Life and Limb

Life and Limb

Perspectives on the
American Civil War

edited by
David Seed,
Stephen C. Kenny
and
Chris Williams

LIVERPOOL UNIVERSITY PRESS

First published 2015 by
Liverpool University Press
4 Cambridge Street
Liverpool
L69 7ZU
UK

www.liverpooluniversitypress.co.uk

British Library Cataloguing-in-Publication data
A British Library CIP record is available

ISBN 978-1-78138-250-9

Typeset by Carnegie Book Production, Lancaster
Printed and bound by CPI Group (UK) Ltd, Croydon, CR0 4YY

Contents

PHOTOGRAPHY

AMPUTATIONS AND PROSTHETIC LIMBS

IN THE FIELD OF BATTLE

POST-WAR NARRATIVES

List of Illustrations

Figures

Plates

Plate 1: Civil War veterans (courtesy National Library of Medicine).

Plate 2: Frontispiece to Louisa May Alcott's *Hospital Sketches* (1869).

Plates 3 and 4: Columbus J. Rush, Private, Co. E, 21st Georgia Volunteers. Amputation of both thighs following shell wounds received at Fort Steadman, Virginia, March 25, 1865. Image reproduced courtesy of the Otis Collection, National Museum of Health and Medicine, Maryland.

Plates 5 and 6: Corporal Charles N. Lapham, 1st Vermont Cavalry. Amputation following wounds from solid shot near Boonsborough, Maryland, July 8, 1863. Image reproduced courtesy of the Otis Collection, National Museum of Health and Medicine, Maryland.

Plates 7 and 8: Carlton Burgan, Private, Co. B, Permall Legion, Maryland Volunteers. Case of osteonecrosis of the jaw subsequent to mercury overdose. Image reproduced courtesy of the Otis Collection, National Museum of Health and Medicine, Maryland.

Plates 9 and 10: Private Rowland Ward, Co. E, 4th New York Heavy Artillery. Cheiloplasty following shell damage to jaw at Ream's Station, Virginia, August 25, 1864. Image reproduced by courtesy of the Otis Collection, National Museum of Health and Medicine, Maryland.

Plate 11: Unknown photographer, 'McPherson's Woods – Wheatfields in which General Reynolds was Shot,' 1863. Digital scan of albumen print. Courtesy Library of Congress.

Plate 12: Andrew J. Russell, 'Rebel Caisson Destroyed by Federal Shells at Fredricksburg, 3 May, 1863.' Digital scan of albumen print. Courtesy Library of Congress.

Plate 13: George N. Barnard, 'Ruins at Charleston, SC,', 1864. Digital scan of albumen print from Barnard's *Photographic Views*, 1866. Courtesy George Eastman House International Museum of Photography and Film.

Plate 14: Unknown photographer(s), 'Surgical photographs [...] prepared under supervision of [...] War Dept., Surgeon General's Office, Army Medical Museum,' c. 1866. Digital scan of album plates. Courtesy Library of Congress.

Plate 15: Willam H. Bell, 'Gunshot Fracture of the Shaft of the Right Femur, United with Great Shortening and Deformity,' 1865. Digital scan of albumen silver print. Courtesy J. Paul Getty Museum.

Acknowledgements

We would like to express our gratitude for the following:

To the School of the Arts and the School of Histories, Languages and Cultures at the University of Liverpool for their support of the entire *Life and Limb* project.

To Blesma, the charity for all serving and ex-Service men and women who have lost limbs or lost the use of limbs or eyes, for their sponsorship of this publication and their support of the *Life and Limb* exhibition.

To Shaun Lowndes for creating the cover artwork for this book.

To Angel Martin, artist and designer of our *Life and Limb* logo.

To Jill Newmark and the National Library of Medicine for permission to use the title *Life and Limb* and the photograph of Civil War veterans.

To the Hanger Clinic for the excerpt from James Edward Hanger's 'Record of Services' and for photographic images.

To the University of North Carolina Press for the excerpt from pp. 20–21 of David Hunter Strother's *A Virginia Yankee in the Civil War*, ed. Cecil D. Eby, Jr. ©1961.

To Mark Farrell for the excerpt from *The Civil War Diary and Letters of Sergeant Henry W. Tisdale*.

To Naomi Roose-Lloyd and the Cultural Affairs section of the U.S. Embassy for their financial support.

Introduction:
Civil War Voices and Views

David Seed (University of Liverpool)

Despite Walt Whitman's doubts that the truth would ever be told about the American Civil War, the historian Louis P. Masur has taken the poet's assertion that 'the real war will never get in the books' as the title for his own anthology, which confirms his assertion that it was a 'written war.'[1] It was a conflict which produced a wealth of accounts ranging from diaries to official reports. While the emphasis in this body of work falls on the wounded and on medical practice, the drama within this writing regularly falls on the interplay between voices, between patient and nurse, observer and participant.

As this collection demonstrates, the boundary between private and public texts blurred repeatedly as participants sought to preserve their records of events. Taking one example from the many, the Southern novelist John Beauchamp Jones served as a clerk in Richmond and published his diary of the war years in 1866. When describing the return of the wounded after successfully repelling an attack, he noted not only the supplies they salvaged: 'There were boxes of lemons, oranges, brandies and wines, and all the luxuries of distant lands which enter the unrestricted ports of the United States. These things were narrated by the pale and bleeding soldiers, who smiled in triumph at their achievement.'[2] Apart from their need of care and attention, the wounded were a source of information which Jones transmitted through his diary. More famously but in a similar spirit, while serving in the hospitals of Washington, DC, Walt Whitman cast himself in the role of mediator between casualties

---

1 Louis P. Masur, ed., *The Real War Will Never Get in the Books* (New York: Oxford University Press, 1993), p. 7.
2 John Beauchamp Jones, *A Rebel War Clark's Diary at the Confederate States Capital* (Philadelphia: J.B. Lippincott, 1866), Vol. 1, Chapter 14.

and public, registering the different stories of the soldiers he encountered. In the last of his 'memoranda' on the war when peace came, he expressed scepticism about whether the 'black infernal background of countless minor scenes and interiors' would ever be conveyed to future generations, making a point which is demonstrated on virtually every page of this anthology.[3] Civil War writing frequently presented a series of small episodes, pictures, anecdotes or case histories, a series of glimpses of a new complex and appalling reality. Whitman's choice of the memorandum or short sketch was strategic in pursuing the vivid particularity of particular cases, for example that of a young soldier from Wisconsin who was fatally wounded in battle. Whitman focuses the pathos of this death in the fact the soldier records in advance of his own death in his diary, writing: *'Today the doctor says I must die – all is over with me – ah, so young to die.'*[4]

Acting on the implication that the soldier articulates his fate more powerfully than could his nurse, Whitman adds no comment to the entry. His brevity contrasts sharply with one of the most elaborate deathbed scenes from the war, that described by Louisa May Alcott in her *Hospital Sketches*. Adopting the persona of Tribulation Periwinkle to place herself within a Puritan tradition of moral commitment, Alcott's account of the death of a blacksmith is elaborately composed as an exemplary episode of pious resignation on the patient's part. John the blacksmith is given his own 'short story,' which contrasts with Alcott's carefully paced narrative of how the news is broken of his impending death. It becomes a moot point who is the protagonist in this account – nurse or patient. As his end approaches John cries out 'for God's sake, give me air!' before he is assimilated into a tableau of death as the coming of sleep. Alcott's description is unusual in its leisured evocation of time and in the implicit self-regard of the narrator. Accounts of nursing tended to be less melodramatic and more anecdotal. Jane Woolsey for one gave thumbnail character sketches of the nurses and officials working with her, sometimes using the descriptive present to convey an immediacy she feared might be lost in the aftermath of the war. Susie Taylor's memoir is angled to redress the preponderance of male accounts she felt were being published. And Sarah Edmonds reduces her role to that of a recording instrument: 'I am simply eyes, ears, hands and feet.'[5]

---

3   Walt Whitman, 'The Real War Will Never Get in the Books,' *Specimen Days & Collect* (Philadelphia: Rees Welsh, 1882–83), p. 80.
4   Whitman, 'DEATH OF A HERO,' *Specimen Days*. Italics in original.
5   Sarah Edmonds, *Nurse and Spy in the Union Army* (Hartford, CT: W.S. Williams, 1865), p. 58.

Whitman's role of mediator was used in a battlefield context by Warren Lee Goss, whose *Recollections of a Private* was probably one of Stephen Crane's sources for *The Red Badge of Courage*. Here Goss uses the generic term 'private' to imply a composite subject. Speaking on behalf of his comrades, in his preface he admits to a certain element of artifice in how he assembled his account, insisting that his title should not be taken too literally: 'the writer has availed himself of the reminiscences of many comrades known by him to be trustworthy. For convenience and to give a greater sense of reality to the descriptions, he has often made use of the first person in chronicling the recollections of his comrades.'[6] Goss's *Recollections* thus dramatizes excerpts from different soldiers' accounts which graphically record the sudden, arbitrary and often grotesque wounds they suffered. The authenticity of his volume comes from these first-hand descriptions. Like Whitman, Goss demonstrates an awareness of the medium he is using to pass on accounts which would otherwise remain unknown. As he admits at the beginning of his preface, 'could their voices have been heard mine would have been silent.'

The role of nurse included writing letters for the wounded or writing to relatives after a death. Jane Woolsey includes within *Hospital Days* samples of this correspondence. For example, she quotes from a letter of 1864, where a soldier's wife describes receiving bad news from Woolsey: 'When I first opened your letter I dare not look at the commencement, but glanced my eye toward the bottom and read, – "Your dear husband had good care during his illness." I tried to think he was better. I jumped up and clapped my hands, and said, – "Oh! It's news from John." I sat down and began to read again until I read, "At half past eight God took him;" when I fell to the floor.'[7] By depicting her reactions through physical acts as if she were observing herself, the correspondent makes her tragedy all the more powerful and Woolsey in effect situates the reader within a chain of correspondence relating us to the fate of her patients in a surprisingly direct way.

Letters were the medium for a number of Civil War memoirs. Spencer Glasgow Welch published *A Confederate Surgeon's Letters to His Wife* perhaps in the hope that family correspondence would displace any expectation of political bias. The preamble to this volume explains that 'personal matter' has been excluded as irrelevant and then reveals that the letters have been condensed and arranged by the surgeon's daughter. In short, the book is the

---

6 Warren Lee Goss, *Recollections of a Private* (New York: Thomas Y. Crowell, 1890), p. iv.
7 Jane Stuart Woolsey, *Hospital Days* (New York: D. Van Nostrand, 1868), p. 144.

result of family collaboration. In contrast, Katherine Wormeley's *The Other Side of War* presents a series of letters mainly to the author's mother, retaining the letter format while editing out the names of recipients. By so doing, she retains the quality of freshness in what were for her novel experiences. Having described a typical day on her first ward, she summarizes the change of shift, or 'watch,' by referring to the moment of composition: 'After dinner other ladies keep the same sort of watch through the afternoon and evening, while we sit on the floor of our state-rooms resting, and perhaps writing letters, as I am doing now.'[8] Here Wormeley contextualizes her memoir within the concrete circumstances of the practices she is recording.

Apart from helping to form records, letters also had an important part to play in the emerging trade in artificial limbs. Promotion of the latter repeatedly included the publication of letters from owners, which clearly served a commercial purpose but which also situated writers within the community of consumers. As Jalynn Olsen Padilla has stated, 'most testimonials to artificial limbs celebrated the men's ability to perform manual labour.'[9] Thus the Cincinnati blacksmith who wrote to B. Frank Palmer in 1864 boasted that he had worn a Palmer leg 'for NINE YEARS, WITHOUT ANY REPAIRS' and claimed that he could work as well as any of his journeymen. Even more importantly, the leg was not immediately visible: 'men have worked beside me every day for months without knowing that I wore an artificial leg.'[10] In such cases the companies are further exploiting the conventional associations of letters with first-hand authenticity. Indeed, they approach the style of advertisements in their use of typography of emphasis through capitals, italics and font size.

In the works just referred to the boundary between personal communication and public text is becoming interestingly blurred and this process can be seen as early as 1863 in Frederick Law Olmsted's *Hospital Transports*. The designer of New York's Central Park, Olmsted was serving as Executive Secretary of the Sanitary Commission at the time and recorded the evacuation of Northern troops from the Virginia peninsula in 1862 with a volume assembled from letters written by nurses and officers participating in the

8   Katherine Wormeley, *The Other Side of War* (Boston: Ticknor and Fields, 1889), p. 27.
9   Jalynn Olsen Padilla, 'Army of "Cripples": Northern Civil War Amputees, Disability and Manhood in Victorian America,' PhD Dissertation, University of Delaware, 2007, pp. 144–45.
10   *The Palmer Arm and Leg, Adopted for the U.S. Army and Navy* (Philadelphia: American Artificial Leg Company, 1865), p. 37.

action. It was exactly the impromptu quality of these letters which gave them their special authenticity. As Olmsted explained, 'they were, for the most part, addressed to intimate friends, with no thought that they could ever go beyond them.' However, he continued, 'they contain thoughts springing from the occasion, and which will serve to fasten pictures of scenes and circumstances with which that service [Hospital Transport] was associated, and which are now historical.'[11] For his memoir, Olmsted preserved the shared authorship by indicating different correspondents through an initial letter. A similar principle of assembly was followed in the *Medical and Surgical History of the War of the Rebellion* (1861–65), which was put together from many field reports.

This history again and again reflects a tension between the anonymous language of medical reports and the voices of the patients themselves. Take the case of Private James Ackerman, who was wounded by gunshot near the elbow joint. The report gives physical details of the wound and notes that the bullet was not found. It continues: 'The patient seemed well and comfortable during the day, but at night was always delirious, frequently screaming out that "the rebels were after him." The arm was placed in an angular tin splint, and dressed with cold water until the inflammation subsided and suppuration became free. He died July 12th, 1862.'[12] The affectless language of clinical physical description suddenly gives way to a glimpse of the patient's subjective life, all the more poignant for being so brief. The night–day contrast hints at a total disconnect between his apparent physical state and his mental well-being, and the latter is signaled through the soldier's voice, with the irony that the convention of free indirect speech has already anticipated his death by shifting his words into the past tense. The affectless language of clinical description is momentarily suspended to evoke the soldier's night-time terrors, and then he is dead, and the language reverts to the physical details of his autopsy. The main point of the report is to supply these details so that the soldier's fate can function as an instructive case. However, the quoted passage briefly opens up the soldier's subjective life, which the report does not – indeed cannot – convey. This tension between the physical and the subjective, between external physical features and internal mental life, inevitably runs through many of these wartime medical reports.

The notion of medical reportage was used as an introductory frame to

11   Frederick Law Olmsted, *Hospital Transports* (Boston: Ticknor and Fields, 1863), p. viii.
12   Joseph K. Barnes, ed. *The Medical and Surgical History of the War of the Rebellion*, Part I, Vol. II (Washington, DC: Government Printing Office, 1870), p. 528.

the 1866 story 'The Case of George Dedlow,' which purports to be taken from the notes of an Indiana surgeon wounded in battle. As a result of this wound, his right arm is amputated. After returning to his regiment, he is wounded yet again, this time losing both legs. As if that wasn't enough, his left arm turns gangrenous and he loses his last limb. While in the 'Stump Hospital' for amputees in Philadelphia, Dedlow engages in amateur (but – it turns out – by no means absurd) observation of the patients' common susceptibility to the 'phantom-limb' phenomenon of imagining sensation in the limbs they have lost. As he is suffering from a perceived reduction of identity, Dedlow is offered consolation by a chaplain and joins a spiritualist circle, where, during a séance, a medium seems to have put him in touch with his lost limbs. The story offsets its bizarre conclusion with perfectly plausible descriptions of the wounded soldiers.

Fast forward to 1871, when Silas Weir Mitchell publishes an article explaining 'phantom limbs' as resulting from severed nerve ends. In his preamble he takes care to distinguish his account from popular impressions and cites (although not by name) the story described above: 'this sketch gave an account of the sensations of men who have lost a limb or limbs, but the author, taking advantage of the freedom accorded to a writer of fiction, described as belonging to this class of sufferers certain psychological states so astounding in their character that he certainly could never have conceived it possible that his humorous sketch, with its absurd conclusion, would for a moment mislead anyone.' He continues: 'Many persons, however, took it as true' and some even organized subscription for the supposed victim.[13] What Mitchell slyly conceals is that the author of the 1866 story was none other than himself! 'The Case of George Dedlow' clearly gained credibility from its skilful imitations of medical discourse and Mitchell's combination in his narrator of the roles of physician and patient draws the reader into the traumatized psychology of an amputee, which was still in the early stages of analysis at the time. The story cuts right across generic distinctions between medical reportage and fiction, hence the misunderstanding by its first readers.

The play of voice against voice might serve practical convenience. At a particular point in one of the illustrator David Hunter Strother's postwar sketches, 'Personal Recollections of the War,' he is speaking to a general. A file of soldiers passes nearby carrying a casualty on a stretcher, at which point the general asks, 'Is that man dead?' The answer comes from Strother himself: '"Dead certainly," I replied. "Observe the ashen hue and rigid pose of the left

<hr>

13   Silas Weir Mitchell, 'Phantom Limbs,' *Lippincott's Magazine of Popular Literature and Science* 8 (1871), p. 564.

hand as it drops below the blanket.'"[14] Whether the exchange actually took place or not is really irrelevant. As we might expect from a graphic artist, Strother only occasionally gives direct speech and uses it here to underline his visual credentials, which are even stronger than the general's, despite the latter's presumable familiarity with battlefields.

Strother was taking part in a postwar mode of writing which could be called sceptical realism. He implicitly turns away from glamorous military spectacle to describe instead the sheer detritus left in the wake of battle. Ambrose Bierce similarly turned away from 'literary bearers of false witness,' who, he implies, betray their subjects.[15] When he opens his 1881 sketch 'What I Saw of Shiloh' with the declaration 'this is a simple story of a battle; such a tale as may be told by a soldier who is no writer to a reader who is no soldier,' he is clearly trying to circumvent conventions of military description. This he does by angling his account through the perspective of an observer-participant who is embedded in the action. One of the main features of battle for Bierce is a reduction of men to a 'mob' acting on a shared need to survive. Battle is presented as a confusing process sweeping men to and fro, arrested by a sudden shocking close-up of a casualty. The process spreads injury alike through trees, livestock and of course humans. The grotesque twist in pieces like 'The Coup de Grace' is the ultimate indignity suffered by casualties as corpses are consumed by swine. Bierce's repeated evocations of chance and irony prevent his sketches from presenting any clear outcomes and show war to be a random sequence of small destructive episodes.

This episodic quality also informs Stephen Crane's *The Red Badge of Courage*, which begins and ends in the midst of war. The novel demonstrates the same tension between individuality and type-quality noted earlier in medical reports, with the protagonist sometimes being named but more often simply referred to as 'the youth.' The novel dramatizes an extended debate over the nature of wounding, where Henry Fleming is the focus of tales of military glory from his reading and other accounts from soldiers. He participates in an intermittent dialogue with his fellow soldiers about the nature of battle and the main irony lies in the fact that his injury is actually the result of a blow from a rifle butt when a soldier refuses to answer his questions. In that sense the protagonist's wound is not the visible sign of valor in battle, as he hoped, but reflects the failure of dialogue and ultimately the impossibility of verbalizing war.

14   David Hunter Strother, 'Personal Recollections of the War: Eighth Paper,' *Harper's New Monthly Magazine* 35 (June–November 1867), p. 289.
15   'A Bivouac of the Dead,' *The Complete Short Stories of Ambrose Bierce* (Lincoln, NE: University of Nebraska Press, 1984), p. 399.

Apart from speech, Henry Fleming constantly struggles to organize his visual impressions into coherent scenes. Once again Crane implies that earlier descriptions of war have no connection with reality and this spirit of visual revisionism runs through much Civil War writing. The flurry of memoirs which followed the armistice shared the common purpose of setting their parts of the record straight, which could be done through images of nursing or through case studies of casualties. David Hunter Strother unusually illustrated his own sketches as well as feeding close visual details into his accounts. The new visual medium which was drawn on throughout the Civil War, however, was photography, used both for medical purposes and for reportage on the conflict, as Mick Gidley explains below. Shirley Samuels has argued that this phenomenon represented the 'first mass distribution of war photography in human history,' continuing: 'for the first time images of live, wounded, and dead bodies from a war were displayed in plate glass windows for the consumption of the viewing public.'[16] She finds a problematic similarity between the photographs in surgeons' notebooks and portrait photographs of the period. Print and visual media alike were used to record and commemorate through the different representational conventions of the time. This collection will introduce the kind of records being produced and also guide the reader towards the ongoing analysis of these works.

A Note on Sources

Full names and titles are given in the body of the text or in the final bibliography. The material excerpted in this collection can be accessed through different websites. A particularly valuable site is the US National Library of Medicine Digital Collections at http://collections.nlm.nih.gov/about.

16   Shirley Samuels, *Facing America* (New York: Oxford University Press, 2004), p. 60.

MEDICAL AND SURGICAL MEMOIRS

Early Experiences in the Field

William Williams Keen (1837–1932) was the first brain surgeon in the United States. He signed up in the army medical corps as Assistant Surgeon in 1861, completing his studies the following year. In the meantime, he served in the aftermath of the first Battle of Bull Run in July 1861, where the Union army suffered heavy casualties. Keen gives a grim account of general lack of medical facilities in the early stages of the war, including his own lack of training. He notes the lack of supplies, recurrence of gangrene, and the shortage of surgeons. Keen studied in Paris and Berlin, going on to become president of the American Medical Association and Professor Surgery.

The following excerpt is from Keen's 'Surgical Reminiscences of the Civil War,' collected in *Addresses and Other Papers* (Philadelphia: W. Saunders, 1905), also in *Transactions of the College of Physicians of Philadelphia* 27 (1905), pp. 95–114.

My first initiation into real warfare was at the First Bull Run. We had marched the day before until after midnight, and were awakened after a brief sleep to the activities of a memorable day in the history of the war. It was an exceedingly hot day, and we marched and halted in the thick dust under a broiling sun until about noon, when my regiment became engaged. Up to that time, and, in fact, during the entire engagement, I never received a single order from either colonel or other officer, medical inspector, the surgeon of my regiment, or anyone else. It was like the days when there was no king in Israel, and every man did that which was right in his own eyes. I did not see the surgeon from the middle of the forenoon. As we approached the battlefield I saw beside a little stream a few surgeons, among whom I knew one, and I asked him what I ought to do, for I was as green as the grass around me as to my duties on the field. My friend Carr, of Rhode Island, suggested that I should turn in there and help, advice which I followed all the more readily because just at that time some of the advance of my own regiment appeared among the wounded. After a time I saw everybody around me packing up and leaving, and upon asking what was the reason was told that they were ordered back to Sedley Springs Church, a mile or more in the rear. Accordingly I went with them, and there in a grove along-side of the road, with no fence to enclose it, stood the little church, perhaps one hundred feet distant from the road. Both inside and outside the church much was on. An operating table was improvised from two hoards laid on two boxes in front of the pulpit. The slightly injured looked down from the gallery upon the industrious surgeons, and a number of kind women from the neighborhood helped to soothe the wounded.

I always have remembered one little illustration of the ignorance even of brigade surgeons who had been hastily appointed at the outbreak of the war. One of the wounded required an amputation at the shoulder-joint, and the operator asked the brigade surgeon to compress the subclavian artery. This he proceeded to do by vigorous pressure applied below the clavicle. With a good deal of hesitation I at last timidly suggested to him that possibly compression above the clavicle would be more efficacious, when, with withering scorn, he informed me that he was pressing in the right place, as was proved by the name of the artery, which was subclavian. I do not remember whether the operator took a hand in this little linguistic discussion or even overheard it. I had my rather grim revenge, happily, not to the serious disadvantage of the patient. When the operator made the internal flap the axillary artery gave one enormous jet of blood, for the subclavian persisted in running where it could be compressed above the clavicle in spite of its name. I caught the artery in the flap, as I had been taught to do by Dr. Winton, and instantly controlled the hemorrhage. Later I was outside the church dressing a man who had a fracture of the humerus from a Minié ball. I was applying a splint and an eight-yard bandage. We were in the wood surrounding the church, perhaps twenty feet back from the road, when suddenly one hundred or more of the soldiers rushed pell-mell down the road from the battlefield crying, 'The rebs are after us!' It did not take more than one positive assertion of this kind to convince the man whose arm I was bandaging that it was time for him to leave, and he broke away from me, rushing for the more distant woods. As he ran four or five yards of the bandage unwound, and I last saw him disappearing in the distance, with this fluttering bobtail bandage flying all abroad.

My experience in this battle is a good illustration of the utter disorganization, or rather want of organization, of our entire army at the beginning of the war.

Case 275

The Medical and Surgical History of the War of the Rebellion, 1861–1865 (MSHWR), prepared under the direction of Joseph K. Barnes, Surgeon-General of the Army, gives statistics assembled from medical reports. Published 1870–88, the volumes include extracts from narratives by individual members of the medical staff. The introduction to Volume 1 states that 'aside from all considerations of a scientific or historical nature, motives of humanity would seem to dictate that the statistics should be presented in the form most likely to render them serviceable as a contribution to our knowledge of the influence of race-peculiarities on disease.' The full text of the history can be found at https://archive.org/details/medicalsurgical22barnrich.

The following text is from *MSHWR* Part II, Vol. II, pp. 90–91.

Lieutenant J.E. Mallet, Adjutant 81st New York, aged 21 years, was wounded at the battle of Cold Harbor, June 3, 1864, by a musket ball, which entered three inches to the left of the umbilicus and made its exit a little to the right of the spinal column [...] This officer, who still survives and holds an important civil office under the Government, has kindly prepared an account of his case, which is peculiarly valuable because of the rarity with which reliable information of the immediate symptoms produced by severe wounds can be obtained. The authenticity of the facts is unquestionable, and, independently of the officer's own statement, is affirmed by the testimony of the medical attendants. 'I was wounded,' says this brave officer, 'at the battle of Cold Harbor, while serving as adjutant of the 81st New York Infantry, or 2nd Oswego Regiment, then with the Army of the Potomac, and attached to the first (Marston's) brigade, first (Brooks's) division, eighteenth (Smith's) Army Corps. It was at about five o'clock in the morning, and in the assault on the enemy's entrenched lines, I was struck. I fell at the distance of about fifteen paces from the works which our men were charging with uncapped pieces. The missile entered my left side. I distinctly remember the sensations experienced upon being hit. I imagined that a cannon ball had struck me on the left hip-bone, that it took a downward course, tearing the intestines in its course, and lodged against the marrow of the right thigh-bone. I fancied I saw sparks of fire, and curtains of cobwebs wet with dew, sparkling in the sun. I heard a monotonous roar as of distant cataracts. I felt my teeth chatter, a rush of blood to my eyes, ears, nose, and to the ends of my fingers and toes. These sensations crowded themselves in the instants in which I struggled to stand, and actually fell forward on my face. As I fell, I experienced another sensation as of a sudden and violent blow on the nape of the neck, and then became completely insensible. I was awakened to consciousness by cheering, and fearing to be trampled by the advancing lines, I made a desperate effort to regain my feet, and doubled up as one with a broken back, with my sword strapped to my right wrist, and the scabbard in the other hand. I dragged myself about forty paces to the right and rear, and entered the skirt of a wood, where I saw men hiding behind trees, which angered me, and I again fell insensible. Later I remember being put on a stretcher by some men of a Massachusetts regiment, and carried some distance to an ambulance. During the day, someone had given me a piece of sponge cake dipped in wine; but it was at once rejected. It rained during the day, and someone covered me with a rubber blanket, which a passer-by presently carried off, and I had the will but not the power to protest. The pain in the wound in the back was intense. I do not recollect distinctly my arrival at the corps hospital; but I recall the visit of Surgeon W.H. Rice, and his exploration of my wound, and his instructions to a friend to take my watch and valuables, and my inference that he considered my case hopeless, and that these mementoes were to be sent home.

'On the afternoon of June 3rd, I was put in an ambulance wagon [...] and taken as far as Bethesda Church, where we stopped overnight. We proceeded on our journey next morning, over very rugged ground. I remember the wounded who could walk, often put their shoulders to the wagon to keep it from upsetting. We arrived at White House Landing, on the York River, late on the afternoon of June 4th. I had suffered much pain from shortness of breath, but was relieved by draughts of water. I was put on a hospital transport and was laid by the side of the deck, where the breeze could reach me; but it seemed to take my breath away instead of restoring it. I was very faint, and Captain Tyler, of my regiment, and others, have since told me that I was regarded as a dead man. I remember nothing further until we reached Alexandria, and finally Washington, where I asked to be taken to Douglas Hospital, but all the wounded were carried off in ambulance wagons, and I thought I was deserted; but finally they brought a stretcher and carried to Armory Square [...] On the morning of June 6th, Medical Inspector Coolidge examined me. From memoranda, made soon afterward, I find that I was frequently unconscious during the next week; but that, on June 12th, I could read the leaded headings of newspapers. On June 15th, I had a distressing pain in the bowels. Gradually my vision improved, and on June 22nd I began to keep my diary. Acting Assistant Surgeon Bowen was attending me. On June 27th, I ate some blackberries, which made me sick, and for the next few days I was feverish and drowsy. On July 1st, I had severe colic. On July 3rd, Surgeon Bliss examined me. On the 5th, I was better, and asked to be sent home. On July 6th, I sat up in an arm-chair. On the 12th, some blackberry seeds were found in the lint removed from the wound in the side. On July 17th, I drank a glass of soda-water, which, in about fifteen minutes, began to bubble out at the orifice in the side, forcing off the adhesive plaster and compresses, and soiling my clothing with a copious foetid discharge of a yellowish color. On July 27th, I was taken on a stretcher to the cars, and rode to New York, and thence on a steamer to Albany, and thence by rail to Oswego, where I arrived on the 29th, and was attended by Dr. C.P.P. Clark, of Fort Ontario. My hospital diet nearly starved me, and I suffered greatly during the dressings. Pieces of shirt and trousers and braces were extracted from the wounds at different times. There was a swelling below the wound, which was very sensitive. Some of the surgeons thought it contained the ball; others that a fragment of the eleventh rib was lodged there. On August 13th, I walked for the first time. On August 26th, there was so much pain in the swelling referred to that a surgical consultation was held, and, on the 28th, Dr. Clark incised the swelling and removed a large button that had been driven in by the ball. On October 1st, I reported at the hospital at Annapolis, and on October 31, 1864, was honorably discharged for wounds received in action, on the recommendation of the board of which General Graham was president. In 1865 my health improved, so that I was able to do clerical duty, and from that time to this (1873) my health has been comparatively good. I am nevertheless subject to pain in the spine at damp seasons. My left side and arm are weak, and, in walking a considerable distance, my left leg becomes lame. It may be proper to add that at the time of receiving the wound I had been fasting for nearly forty-eight hours.'

The principal facts above recited in a connected form, appear, separately, in the reports of Surgeons W.H. Rice, 81st New York, H. P. Porter, 10th Connecticut, Acting Assistant Surgeon C.H. Bowen, and Surgeon B.A. Vanderkieft, U.S.V. Dr. Bowen remarks that the evidence of extensive destruction of the wall of the descending colon was conclusive, and that a spinous process of a vertebra was probably fractured. The evidence of the intestinal lesion consisted in a copious fæcal discharge from the wound, which persisted for several weeks, while the patient was at Armory Square. Mr. Mallet received the brevet of Major of United States Volunteers for gallantry.

ACCOUNTS OF NURSING

With the US Sanitary Commission:
On the Hospital Boat *Wilson Small*

Katherine Prescott Wormeley (1830–1908) was born in Ipswich, England, the daughter of a naval officer. She had settled in the United States by the outbreak of war and served as a nurse in the US Sanitary Commission, an organization of volunteers whose activities supplemented the Medical Division of the Union army, which grew, in Wormeley's words, into 'a great machine running side by side with the Medical Bureau wherever the armies went' (*The Other Side of War*, p. 10). Its members organized 'Sanitary Fairs' to raise funds and supplies. Wormeley served mainly on hospital boats and later published letters recording her impressions. She also published numerous translations of French literary works.

The following text is from Wormeley's *The Other Side of War: Letters from Headquarters during the Peninsula Campaign* (Boston: Ticknor and Fields, 1889), in 1898 re-titled *The Cruel Side of War*.

May 13th 1862. Yesterday I came on board this boat, where there are thirty very bad cases – four or five amputations. One poor fellow, a lieutenant in the Thirty-second New York Volunteers, shot through the knee, and enduring more than mortal agony; a fair-haired boy of seventeen, shot through the lungs, every breath he draws hissing through the wound; another man, a poet, with seven holes in him, but irrepressibly poetic and very comical. He dictated to me last night a foolscap sheet full of poetry composed for the occasion. His appearance as he sits up in bed, swathed in a nondescript garment or poncho, constructed for him by Miss Whetten out of an old green table-cloth, is irresistibly funny. There is also a captain of the Sixteenth New York Volunteers, mortally wounded while leading his company against a regiment. He is said to measure six feet seven inches – and I believe it, looking at him as he lies there on a cot, pieced out at the foot with two chairs.

I took my first actual watch last night; and this morning I feel the same ease about the work which yesterday I was surprised to see in others. We begin the day by getting them all washed, and freshened up, and breakfasted. Then the surgeons and dressers make their rounds, open the wounds, apply the remedies, and replace the bandages. This is an awful hour; I sat with my fingers in my ears this morning. When it is over, we go back to the men and put the ward in order once more, re-making several of the beds, and giving clean handkerchiefs with a little cologne or bay-water on them – so prized in the sickening atmosphere of wounds. We sponge the bandages over the wounds constantly – which alone carries us round from cot to cot almost without stopping, except to talk to some, read to others, or write letters for them; occasionally giving medicine or brandy, etc., according to order. Then comes dinner, which we serve ourselves, feeding those who can't feed themselves. After that we go off duty, and get first washed and then fed ourselves, our dinner-table being the top of an old stove, with slices of bread for plates, fingers for knives and forks, and carpet-bags for chairs – all this because everything available is being used for our poor fellows. After dinner other ladies keep the same sort of watch through the afternoon and evening, while we sit on the floor of our state-rooms resting, and perhaps writing letters, as I am doing now.

Evacuation from Virginia, 1862

Frederick Law Olmsted (1822–1903) was the designer of Central Park in New York and other parks in the United States. During the war he served as leader of the Sanitary Commission. The following is from Olmsted's *Hospital Transports. A Memoir of the Embarkation of the Sick and Wounded from the Peninsula of Virginia in the Summer of 1862* (Boston: Ticknor and Fields, 1863).

The *Spaulding* is bunked in every hole and corner, and is a most inconvenient ship for carrying sick men, everything above decks running to first-classing, and everything below to steerage. The last hundred patients were put on board, to relieve the over-crowded shore hospital, late last night. Though these night scenes on the hospital ships are part of our daily living, a fresh eye would find them dramatic. We are awakened in the dead of night by a sharp steam-whistle, and soon after feel ourselves clawed by the little tugs on either side of our big ship – and at once the process of taking on hundreds of men, many of them crazed with fever, begins. There's the bringing of the stretchers up the side ladder between the two boats, the stopping at the head of it, where the names and home addresses of all who can speak are written down, and their knapsacks and little treasures numbered and stacked; – then the placing of the stretchers on the platform, the row of anxious faces above and below decks, the lantern held over the hold, the word given to 'Lower!' the slow-moving ropes and pulleys, the arrival at the bottom, the turning down of the anxious faces, the lifting out of the sick man, and the lifting him into his bed; – and then the sudden change from cold, hunger, and friendlessness, to positive comfort and satisfaction, winding up with his invariable verdict – if he can speak – 'This is just like home!'

Hospital Routine

Jane Woolsey (1830–1891) was living in New York at the outbreak of war. She participated in the Women's Central Relief Association, a precursor of the US Sanitary Commission, and in 1861–62 visited a number of New York hospitals as a member of the Women's Auxiliary Commission. In 1863, while training in Rhode Island, she was invited to serve as supervisor of the Fairfax Seminary Hospital in Alexandria, Virginia.

The following excerpts are from Woolsey's *Hospital Days: Reminiscence of a Civil War Nurse* (New York: D. Van Nostrand, 1868). *Hospital Days* gives a series of vignettes showing the day-to-day routine activities of a nurse during the war: dietary measures, visits by the Superintendent, chaplain's visits, etc. She noted that 'the whole air and tone of a hospital ward change and rise after a few days of a woman's presence' (p. 43). Her record includes accounts of conversations with patients and sample letters from family members of deceased patients.

[from 'Superintendent's Day']

The woman-nurse in each little ward-room receives her tray or trays, having her china plates and cups, her knives and forks and tumblers, set out in order beforehand; divides the food according to a duplicate of the ward return hanging over her table, and the men-nurses carry it about. She follows immediately down the ward, helps and feeds those who are unable to help themselves, and sees that all have enough. If anything goes wrong, she is directed to send word at once to the Superintendent. She has means of heating over any simple thing if the patient does not incline to it at the fixed hour. A sick man will often take his food nicely if he may have his own time about it, and does not feel himself under observation. In critical cases a fresh ration is prepared instead of the rechauffe. The small special blanks (F) are meant for these and all other cases of emergency; or the woman-nurse can have anything urgently needed at the moment, by sending her own written request for it. Extra rations of one or two articles – such as beef-tea, oysters, eggs – are always on hand in the kitchen. The Government ration is so generous that when honestly used there is almost always margin enough for extra calls without extra requisitions for raw material. The commissary steward, however, is required by the Surgeon in Charge to keep some trustworthy person in the storehouse ready at all times to fill such requisitions.

The Superintendent follows in the wake of the diet car. Such is the celerity with which the Defenders, even when ill, swallow their food, it is impossible to be in more than one or two wards while eating is actually going on. But by beginning at a different and unexpected ward and meal every day, the objects of an inspection are pretty well secured. 'Was the gruel right?' 'Did you get a full tumbler of punch?' 'You are tired of the beef-tea? Grumble as much as you like.' 'But I don't want to grumble; I aint got no complaints to make – only,' – aside to G – 'I'd as lief see the devil coming up the ward as that beef-tea!'

[from 'Women-Nurses']

Was the system of Women-nurses in hospitals a failure? There never was any system. That the presence of hundreds of individual women as nurses in hospitals was neither an intrusion nor a blunder, let the multitude of their – unsystematized – labours and achievements testify. So far as I know, the experiment of a compact, general organization was never fairly tried. Hospital nurses were of all sorts, and came from various sources of supply; volunteers paid or unpaid; soldiers' wives and sisters who had come to see their friends, and remained without any clear commission or duties ; women sent by State agencies and aid societies ; women assigned by the General Superintendent of Nurses ; sometimes, as in a case I knew of, the wife or daughter of a medical officer drawing the rations, but certainly not doing the work of a 'laundress.' These women were set adrift in a hospital, eight to twenty of them, for the most part slightly educated, without training or discipline, without company organi-zation or officers, so to speak, of their own, 'reporting' to the surgeons, or in the case of persons assigned by her, to the General Superintendent, which is very much, in a small way, as if Private Robinson should 'report' to General Grant.

[...]

Mrs. A---- had 'come out,' she told me 'to *cresh* the rebellion,' which she conceived she could best do by distributing inordinate quantities of what she called 'sanitary jel.' She had a difference with Mrs. C---, who considered pickled cucumbers the proper weapons to use against the enemies of the country.

[...]

Miss D--- was an excellent little creature, gentle-mannered, delicate, tremulous, full of intense and indignant patriotism. Night and day found her unflagging in her place. Watch had to be kept over her lest she should never get proper food or rest. She could not work by rule or method. She lost the law in the exceptions. She took what she thought 'short cuts,' and hand-to-mouth ways of doing what systematic effort would have accomplished in half the time. She was full of goodness and devotion. When she was not at a patient's pillow she was hurrying eagerly to the storeroom to collect comforts and tell the abuses and atrocities she had seen. She thought all military restriction atrocious. She wanted 'to go and see Mr. Lincoln about it.' Her health gave way before the end of the war and she went home. We were very sorry to part with her. I am afraid the generous heart that beat so fast is scarcely beating now.

[...]

Miss S--- was a German who had followed a relative to the Hospital, and asked for employment as a nurse. She had her virtues and her uses, chief of which was interpreting between the ward surgeon and the German patients. She was a famous knitter of nice woollen socks. She supplied and repaired the whole ward. But she could not resist feeding her 'browthers' clandestinely, with the delicacies of their native land, made in the nurses' mess kitchen. One of these was a warm and washy beverage called 'beer-soup,' and another was an anonymous mixture of something like glue, cabbage, and 'pot-scrapings.' We rather winked at the beer-soup, for beer in any shape is such a comfort to the brave Teuton, but the pasty compound was too much for professors of Special Diet, to say nothing of exasperated surgeons.

[from 'In the Store-Room']

The Surgeon in Charge believed in Food as a curative agent. He ordered it in large quantities for men who had suffered severe operations ; and our experience certainly justified his theories, for these men got well, went home, had the small-pox, married their sweethearts, set up shops and wrote back for all our photographs to hang up in them. Vandenhoff, Sawyer, Tyler, McClain, Ripley, Brown, Gregg; a host of names suggest themselves. All these took large quantities of beef-essence, and brandy-and-eggs to the extent of one half-pint tumbler full every two hours.

Sergeant G. exsection of shoulder, Dec. 25th, 1863, took oyster soup, chicken soup, eggs at every meal prepared in different ways, besides forty-eight ounces of egg-nog and two to three bottles of porter every day for several weeks. He then came under the ordinary Special Diet table and took roast beef, vegetables and pudding with one or two pints of milk-punch every day. Early in March he was able to travel and was discharged and went to Philadelphia, where he was promised a good place as watchman. The Sergeant enjoyed all his meals and showed no failure and certainly no delicacy of appetite, as he had an immense craving for an article, furnished he declared, in perfection only by the Philadelphia markets, the intestines of a hog compounded with spices. To gratify him inquiries were made, but this savoury dish could not be obtained.

A Death in the Ward

Louisa May Alcott (1832–1888) was a member of a famous reformist family and was beginning to establish herself as a writer when war broke out. The number of female nurses increased during 1862 under the direction of Dorothea Dix, a family friend of the Alcotts. Alcott herself served in the Georgetown Union Hotel Hospital, just outside Washington, DC, from December 1862 to January 1863, when she fell ill with typhoid pneumonia and was invalided out of the service.

Alcott's *Hospital Sketches* was first published in the abolitionist journal *Boston Commonwealth* from May to June 1863, and was published in book form in 1863 (Boston: James Redpath). Five cents from every copy sold was donated by the publisher to orphans made fatherless or homeless by the war. In her postscript, Alcott criticized the casual disposal of the dead, the callous attitude of some doctors, and also declared: 'Since the appearance of these hasty Sketches, I have heard from several of my comrades at the Hospital; and their approval assures me that I have not let sympathy and fancy run away with me, as that lively team is apt to do when harnessed to a pen,' concluding: '[T]he next hospital I enter will, I hope, be one for the colored regiments, as they seem to be proving their right to the admiration and kind offices of their white relations, who owe them so large a debt, a little part of which I shall be so proud to pay.'

Alcott narrated her sketches through the persona of Tribulation Periwinkle, who declares her commitment to service in the opening line: 'I want something to do.' The later edition of the book, *Hospital Sketches and Camp and Fireside Stories* (Boston: Roberts Brothers, 1869), carried the famous frontispiece reproduced in this volume (see Plate 2). The image shows a hospital scene presided over by a portrait of Lincoln, headed by the motto 'In God We Trust' (which first appeared on coins in 1864), uniting the union cause with Christianity. The patient's eyes are raised (in piety?), the nurse's solicitously directed on the patient.

Alcott's account of the death of Virginia blacksmith John Suhre (in the following excerpt from the sketch 'A Night') contrasts with most other excerpts selected here in its detailed account of his stoical piety, which Alcott uses polemically against the casual treatment of war casualties she witnessed in the hospital. The description is presented as an exemplum, no doubt impractical in battlefield contexts, of spiritual as well as physical care. Through the figure of John, Alcott tacitly invests the Union cause with a unique spiritual authority.

Ednah Dow Cheney's *Louisa May Alcott, Her Life, Letters, and Journals* (Boston: Little, Brown, and Company, 1924) contains excerpts from Alcott's original journals. See also Kathleen Krull, *Louisa May's Battle: How the Civil War Led to 'Little Women'* (London: Walker Childrens, 2013).

My ward was now divided into three rooms; and, under favour of the matron, I had managed to sort out the patients in such a way that I had what I called, 'my duty room,' my 'pleasure room,' and my 'pathetic room,' and worked for each in a different way. One, I visited, armed with a dressing tray, full of rollers, plasters, and pins; another, with books, flowers, games, and gossip; a third, with teapots, lullabies, consolation, and sometimes, a shroud.

[...]

The next night, as I went my rounds with Dr. P., I happened to ask which man in the room probably suffered most; and, to my great surprise, he glanced at John:

'Every breath he draws is like a stab; for the ball pierced the left lung, broke a rib, and did no end of damage here and there; so the poor lad can find neither forgetfulness nor ease, because he must lie on his wounded back or suffocate. It will be a hard struggle, and a long one, for he possesses great vitality; but even his temperate life can't save him; I wish it could.'

'You don't mean he must die, Doctor?'

'Bless you there's not the slightest hope for him; and you'd better tell him so before long; women have a way of doing such things comfortably, so I leave it to you. He won't last more than a day or two, at furthest.'

I could have sat down on the spot and cried heartily, if I had not learned the wisdom of bottling up one's tears for leisure moments. Such an end seemed very hard for such a man, when half a dozen worn out, worthless bodies round him, were gathering up the remnants of wasted lives, to linger on for years perhaps, burdens to others, daily reproaches to themselves. The army needed men like John, dearest, brave, and faithful; fighting for liberty and justice with both heart and hand, true soldiers of the Lord. I could not give him up so soon, or think with any patience of so excellent a nature robbed of its fulfillment, and blundered into eternity by the rashness or stupidity of those at whose hands so many lives may be required. It was an easy thing for Dr. P. to say: 'Tell him he must die,' but a cruelly hard thing to do, and by no means as 'comfortable' as he politely suggested. I had not the heart to do it then, and privately indulged the hope that some change for the better might take place, in spite of gloomy prophesies; so, rendering my task unnecessary. A few minutes later, as I came in again, with fresh rollers, I saw John sitting erect, with no one to support him, while the surgeon dressed his back. I had never hitherto seen it done; for, having simpler wounds to attend to, and knowing the fidelity of the attendant, I had left John to him, thinking it might be more agreeable and safe; for both strength and experience were needed in his case. I had forgotten that the strong man might long for the gentle tendance of a woman's hands, the sympathetic magnetism of a woman's presence, as well as the feebler souls about him. The Doctor's words caused me to reproach myself with neglect, not of any real duty perhaps, but of those little cares and kindnesses that solace homesick spirits, and make the heavy hours pass easier. John looked lonely and forsaken just then, as he sat with bent head, hands folded on his knee, and no outward sign of suffering, till, looking nearer, I saw great tears roll down and drop upon the floor. It was a new sight there; for, though I had seen many suffer, some swore, some groaned, most endured silently, but none wept. Yet it did not seem weak, only very touching, and straightway my fear vanished, my heart opened wide and took him in, as, gathering the bent head in my arms, as freely as if he had been a little child, I said, 'Let me help you bear it, John.'

Never, on any human countenance, have I seen so swift and beautiful a look of gratitude, surprise and comfort, as that which answered me more eloquently than the whispered –

'Thank you, ma'am, this is right good! this is what I wanted!'

'Then why not ask for it before?'

'I didn't like to be a trouble; you seemed so busy, and I could manage to get on alone.'

'You shall not want it any more, John.'

Nor did he; for now I understood the wistful look that sometimes followed me, as I went out, after a brief pause beside his bed, or merely a passing nod, while busied with those who seemed to need me more than he, because more urgent in their demands; now I knew that to him, as to so many, I was the poor substitute for mother, wife, or sister, and in his eyes no stranger, but a friend who hitherto had seemed neglectful; for, in his modesty, he had never guessed the truth. This was changed now; and, through the tedious operation of probing, bathing, and dressing his wounds, he leaned against me, holding my hand fast, and, if pain wrung further tears from him, no one saw them fall but me. When he was laid down again, I hovered about him, in a remorseful state of mind that would not let me rest, till I had bathed his face, brushed his 'bonny brown hair,' set all things smooth about him, and laid a knot of heath and heliotrope on his clean pillow. While doing this, he watched me with the satisfied expression I so liked to see; and when I offered the little nosegay, held it carefully in his great hand, smoothed a ruffled leaf or two, surveyed and smelt it with an air of genuine delight, and lay contentedly regarding the glimmer of the sunshine on the green. Although the manliest man among my forty, he said, 'Yes, ma'am,' like a little boy; received suggestions for his comfort with the quick smile that brightened his whole face; and now and then, as I stood tidying the table by his bed, I felt him softly touch my gown, as if to assure himself that I was there. Anything more natural and frank I never saw, and found this brave John as bashful as brave, yet full of excellencies and fine aspirations, which, having no power to express themselves in words, seemed to have bloomed into his character and made him what he was.

After that night, an hour of each evening that remained to him was devoted to his ease or pleasure. He could not talk much, for breath was precious, and he spoke in whispers; but from occasional conversations, I gleaned scraps of private history which only added to the affection and respect I felt for him. Once he asked me to write a letter, and as I settled pen and paper, I said, with an irrepressible glimmer of feminine curiosity, 'Shall it be addressed to wife, or mother, John?'

'Neither, ma'am; I've got no wife, and will write to mother myself when I get better. Did you think I was married because of this?' he asked, touching a plain ring he wore, and often turned thoughtfully on his finger when he lay alone.

'Partly that, but more from a settled sort of look you have; a look which young men seldom get until they marry.'

'I didn't know that; but I'm not so very young, ma'am, thirty in May, and have been what you might call settled this ten years; for mother's a widow, I'm the oldest child she has, and it wouldn't do for me to marry until Lizzy has a home of her own, and Laurie's learned his trade; for we're not rich, and I must be father to the children and husband to the dear old woman, if I can.'

'No doubt but you are both, John; yet how came you to go to war, if you felt so? Wasn't enlisting as bad as marrying?'

'No, ma'am, not as I see it, for one is helping my neighbor, the other pleasing myself. I went because I couldn't help it. I didn't want the glory or the pay; I wanted the right thing done, and people kept saying the men who were in earnest ought to fight. I was in earnest, the Lord knows! but I held off as long as I could, not knowing which was my duty; mother saw the case, gave me her ring to keep me steady, and said "Go": so I went.'

A short story and a simple one, but the man and the mother were portrayed better than pages of fine writing could have done it.

'Do you ever regret that you came, when you lie here suffering so much?'

'Never, ma'am; I haven't helped a great deal, but I've shown I was willing to give my life, and perhaps I've got to; but I don't blame anybody, and if it was to do over again, I'd do it. I'm a little sorry I wasn't wounded in front; it looks cowardly to be hit in the back, but I obeyed orders, and it don't matter in the end, I know.'

Poor John! it did not matter now, except that a shot in the front might have spared the long agony in store for him. He seemed to read the thought that troubled me, as he spoke so hopefully when there was no hope, for he suddenly added:

'This is my first battle; do they think it's going to be my last?'

'I'm afraid they do, John.'

It was the hardest question I had ever been called upon to answer; doubly hard with those clear eyes fixed on mine, forcing a truthful answer by their own truth. He seemed a little startled at first, pondered over the fateful fact a moment, then shook his head, with a glance at the broad chest and muscular limbs stretched out before him:

'I'm not afraid, but it's difficult to believe all at once. I'm so strong it don't seem possible for such a little wound to kill me.'

[The nurse later returns to his bedside]

As I went in, John stretched out both hands:

'I knew you'd come! I guess I'm moving on, ma'am.'

He was; and so rapidly that, even while he spoke, over his face I saw the grey veil falling that no human hand can lift. I sat down by him, wiped the drops from his forehead, stirred the air about him with the slow wave of a fan, and waited to help him die. He stood in sore need of help – and I could do so little; for, as the doctor had foretold, the strong body rebelled against death, and fought every inch of the way, forcing him to draw each breath with a spasm, and clench his hands with an imploring look, as if he asked, 'How long must I endure this, and be still!' For hours he suffered dumbly, without a moment's respire, or a moment's murmuring; his limbs grew cold, his face damp, his lips white, and, again and again, he tore the covering off his breast, as if the lightest weight added to his agony; yet through it all, his eyes never lost their perfect serenity, and the man's soul seemed to sit therein, undaunted by the ills that vexed his flesh.

One by one, the men woke, and round the room appeared a circle of pale faces and watchful eyes, full of awe and pity; for, though a stranger, John was beloved by all. Each man there had wondered at his patience, respected his piety, admired his fortitude, and now lamented his hard death; for the influence of an upright nature had made itself deeply felt, even in one little week. Presently, the Jonathan who so loved this comely David, came creeping from his bed for a last look and word. The kind soul was full of trouble, as the choke in his voice, the grasp of his hand, betrayed; but there were no tears, and the farewell of the friends was the more touching for its brevity.

'Old boy, how are you?' faltered the one.

'Most through, thank heaven!' whispered the other.

'Can I say or do anything for you anywheres?'

'Take my things home, and tell them that I did my best.'

'I will! I will!'

'Good bye, Ned.'

'Good bye, John, good bye!'

They kissed each other, tenderly as women, and so parted, for poor Ned could not stay to see his comrade die. For a little while, there was no sound in the room but the drip of water, from a stump or two, and John's distressful gasps, as he slowly breathed his life away. I thought him nearly gone, and had just laid down the fan, believing its help to be no longer needed, when suddenly he rose up in his bed, and cried out with a bitter cry that broke the silence, sharply startling every one with its agonized appeal:

'For God's sake, give me air!'

It was the only cry pain or death had wrung from him, the only boon he had asked; and none of us could grant it, for all the airs that blew were useless now. Dan flung up the window. The first red streak of dawn was warming the grey east, a herald of the coming sun; John saw it, and with the love of light which lingers in us to the end, seemed to read in it a sign of hope of help, for, over his whole face there broke that mysterious expression, brighter than any smile, which often comes to eyes that look their last. He laid himself gently down; and, stretching out his strong right arm, as if to grasp and bring the blessed air to his lips in a fuller flow, lapsed into a merciful unconsciousness, which assured us that for him suffering was forever past. He died then; for, though the heavy breaths still tore their way up for a little longer, they were but the waves of an ebbing tide that beat unfelt against the wreck, which an immortal voyager had deserted with a smile. He never spoke again, but to the end held my hand close, so close that when he was asleep at last, I could not draw it away. Dan helped me, warning me as he did so that it was unsafe for dead and living flesh to lie so long together; but though my hand was strangely cold and stiff, and four white marks remained across its back, even when warmth and colour had returned elsewhere, I could not but be glad that, through its touch, the presence of human sympathy, perhaps, had lightened that hard hour.

Nurse and Spy

Sarah Emma Edmonds (1841–1898) was born in New Brunswick, Canada and in the 1850s emigrated to the United States because of her 'insatiable thirst for education,' in her own words. On the outbreak of war she organized a door-to-door appeal for hospital supplies from the householders of Washington. She enlisted in the Union army dressed as a man and saw a number of battles at first hand. Apart from serving as a field nurse, she joined the Union secret service after a number of tests including a phrenological examination to check her 'organs of secretiveness.' Disguised as an African American 'contraband,' she passed behind Southern lines to report on their fortifications, troop dispositions, etc. A further expedition involved disguising herself as an Irish peddler. She also served as a Union 'detective,' tracking and exposing spies in the Northern army. Fair Oaks, Virginia, was the site of two battles in 1862 during the Peninsula Campaign.

The following is taken from Edmonds' *Nurse and Spy in the Union Army: Comprising the Adventures and Experiences of a Woman in Hospitals, Camps, and Battle-Fields* (Hartford, CT: W.S. Williams, etc. 1865). First published as *The Female Spy of the Union Army* (Boston: De Wolfe, Fiske, 1864).

The hospitals in Washington, Alexandria and Georgetown were crowded with wounded, sick, discouraged soldiers. That extraordinary march from Bull Run, through rain, mud, and chagrin, did more toward filling the hospitals than did the battle itself. I found Mrs. B. in a hospital, suffering from typhoid fever, while Chaplain B. was looking after the temporal and spiritual wants of the men with his usual energy and sympathy. He had many apologies to offer 'for running away with my horse,' as he termed it. There were many familiar faces missing, and it required considerable time to ascertain the fate of my friends. Many a weary walk I had from one hospital to another to find some missing one who was reported to have been sent to such and such a hospital [...].

Measles, dysentery and typhoid fever were the prevailing diseases after the retreat. After spending several days in visiting the different hospitals, looking after personal friends, and writing letters for the soldiers who were not able to write for themselves, I was regularly installed in one of the general hospitals. I will here insert an extract from my journal: 'Aug. 3d, 1861. Georgetown, D.C. Have been on duty all day. John C. is perfectly wild with delirium, and keeps shouting at the top of his voice some military command, or, when vivid recollections of the battle-field come to his mind, he enacts a pantomime of the terrible strife – he goes through the whole manual of arms as correctly as if he were in the ranks; and as he, in imagination, loads and fires in quick succession, the flashing of his dying eye and the nervous vigor of his trembling hands give fearful interest to the supposed encounter with the enemy. When we tell him the enemy has retreated, he persists in pursuing; and throwing his arms wildly around him he shouts to his men – "Come on and fight while there is a rebel left in Virginia!" My friend Lieut. M. is extremely weak and nervous, and the wild ravings of J.C. disturb him exceedingly. I requested Surgeon P. to have him removed to a more quiet ward, and received in reply – "This is the most quiet ward in the whole building." There are five hundred patients here who require constant attention, and not half enough nurses to take care of them.

'Oh, what an amount of suffering I am called to witness every hour and every moment. There is no cessation, and yet it is strange that the sight of all this suffering and death does not affect me more. I am simply eyes, ears, hands and feet. It does seem as if there is a sort of stoicism granted for such occasions. There are great, strong men dying all around me, and while I write there are three being carried past the window to the dead room. This is an excellent hospital – everything is kept in good order, and the medical officers are skilful, kind and attentive.'

[...]

On the evening of the same day in which the victory was won I visited what was then, and is still called, the 'hospital tree,' near Fair Oaks. It was an immense tree under whose shady, extended branches the wounded were carried and laid down to await the stimulant, the opiate, or the amputating knife, as the case might require. The ground around that tree for several acres in extent was literally drenched with human blood, and the men were laid so close together that there was no such thing as passing between them; but each one was removed in their turn as the surgeons could attend to them. I witnessed there some of the most heart-rending sights it is possible for the human mind to conceive.

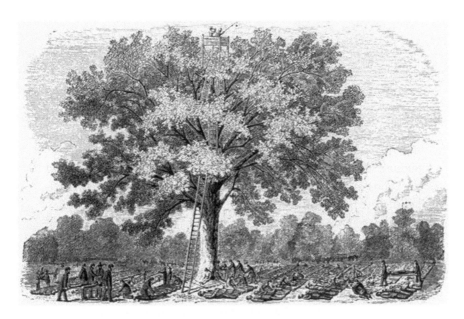

Figure 1: The hospital tree

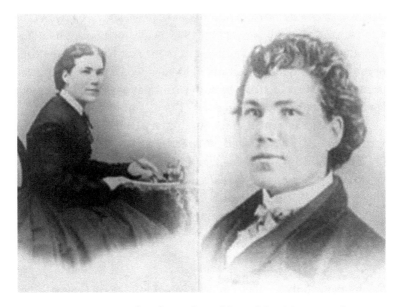

Figure 2: Sarah Edmonds and 'Franklin Thompson'

Front-line Nursing

The daughter of Georgia slaves, Susie King Taylor (1848–1912) served as nurse and teacher in the Union army without pay. In 1862 she became the first African American teacher to freed slaves on St. Simon's Island, Georgia, and married an African American officer in the Union army, where she was the first black nurse to serve. Through her life she held a number of teaching posts.

The below excerpt is taken from Chapter 6 ('On Morris and Other Islands') of Taylor's *Reminiscences of My Life in Camp with the 33d United States Coloured Troops, Late 1st S.C. Volunteers*, written in the 1890s, published in 1902. Fort Wagner on Morris Island was a heavily fortified location for guarding Charleston Harbour.

Mary A. Gardner Holland, who saw nursing experience herself, produced a commemorative collection in *Our Army Nurses. Interesting Sketches, Addresses and Photographs of nearly One Hundred of the Noble Women who Served in Hospitals and on Battlefields during Our Civil War* (Boston: B. Williams, 1895). She made no bones about her patriotic purpose, declaring: 'It seems to me that had I died battling for my country's honour, that my right hand would almost leap from its entombed dust to strike back the arm that would dare drag our flag from its high standard of glory' (17).

For further information see Susan-Mary Grant, 'To Bind Up the Nation's Wounds: Women and the American Civil War', in Kleinberg, S.J., Boris, E., Ruiz, V.L., eds, *The Practice of US Women's History: Narratives, Intersections, and Dialogues* (New Brunswick, NJ: Rutgers University Press, 2007), pp. 106–25.

Fort Wagner being only a mile from our camp, I went there two or three times a week, and would go up on the ramparts to watch the gunners send their shells into Charleston (which they did every fifteen minutes), and had a full view of the city from that point. Outside of the fort were many skulls lying about; I have often moved them one side out of the path. The comrades and I would have quite a debate as to which side the men fought on. Some thought they were the skulls of our boys; others thought they were the enemy's; but as there was no definite way to know, it was never decided which could lay claim to them. They were a gruesome sight, those fleshless heads and grinning jaws, but by this time I had become accustomed to worse things and did not feel as I might have earlier in my camp life.

It seems strange how our aversion to seeing suffering is overcome in war – how we are able to see the most sickening sights, such as men with their limbs blown off and mangled by the deadly shells, without a shudder; and instead of turning away, how we hurry to assist in alleviating their pain, bind up their wounds, and press the cool water to their parched lips, with feelings only of sympathy and pity.

About the first of June, 1864, the regiment was ordered to Folly Island, staying there until the latter part of the month, when it was ordered to Morris Island. We landed on Morris Island between June and July, 1864. This island was a narrow strip of sandy soil, nothing growing on it but a few bushes and shrubs. The camp was one mile from the boat landing, called Pawnell Landing, and the landing one mile from Fort Wagner.

Colonel Higginson had left us in May of this year, on account of wounds received at Edisto. All the men were sorry to lose him. They did not want him to go, they loved him so. He was kind and devoted to his men, thoughtful for their comfort, and we missed his genial presence from the camp.

The regiment under Colonel Trowbridge did garrison duty, but they had troublesome times from Fort Gregg, on James Island, for the rebels would throw a shell over on our island every now and then. Finally orders were received for the boys to prepare to take Fort Gregg, each man to take 150 rounds of cartridges, canteens of water, hard-tack, and salt beef. This order was sent three days prior to starting, to allow them to be in readiness. I helped as many as I could to pack haversacks and cartridge boxes.

The fourth day, about five o'clock in the afternoon, the call was sounded, and I heard the first sergeant say, 'Fall in, boys, fall in,' and they were not long obeying the command. Each company marched out of its street, in front of their colonel's headquarters, where they rested 1862. That same year he founded the Army Medical Museum, for half an hour, as it was not dark enough, and they did not want the enemy to have a chance to spy their movements. At the end of this time the line was formed with the 103d New York (white) in the rear, and off they started, eager to get to work. It was quite dark by the time they reached Pawnell Landing. I have never forgotten the good-byes of that day, as they left camp. Colonel Trowbridge said to me as he left, 'Good-by, Mrs. King, take care of yourself if you don't see us again.' I went with them as far as the landing, and watched them until they got out of sight, and then I returned to the camp. There was no one at camp but those left on picket and a few disabled soldiers, and one woman, a friend of mine, Mary Shaw, and it was lonesome and sad, now that the boys were gone, some never to return.

Mary Shaw shared my tent that night, and we went to bed, but not to sleep, for the fleas nearly ate us alive. We caught a few, but it did seem, now that the men were gone, that every flea in camp had located my tent, and caused us to vacate. Sleep being out of the question, we sat up the remainder of the night.

About four o'clock, July 2, the charge was made. The firing could be plainly heard in camp. I hastened down to the landing and remained there until eight o'clock that morning. When the wounded arrived, or rather began to arrive, the first one brought in was Samuel Anderson of our company. He was badly wounded. Then others of our boys, some with their legs off, arm gone, foot off, and wounds of all kinds imaginable. They had to wade through creeks and marshes, as they were discovered by the enemy and shelled very badly. A number of the men were lost, some got fastened in the mud and had to cut off the legs of their pants, to free themselves. The 103d New York suffered the most, as their men were very badly wounded.

My work now began. I gave my assistance to try to alleviate their sufferings. I asked the doctor at the hospital what I could get for them to eat. They wanted soup, but that I could not get; but I had a few cans of condensed milk and some turtle eggs, so I thought I would try to make some custard. I had doubts as to my success, for cooking with turtle eggs was something new to me, but the adage has it, 'Nothing ventured, nothing done,' so I made a venture and the result was a very delicious custard. This I carried to the men, who enjoyed it very much. My services were given at all times for the comfort of these men. I was on hand to assist whenever needed. I was enrolled as company laundress, but I did very little of it, because I was always busy doing other things through camp, and was employed all the time doing something for the officers and comrades.

'The Mute Look that Rolls and Moves': Walt Whitman's Civil War

Robert Leigh Davis (Wittenberg University)

Attention is the rarest and purest form of generosity.

– Simone Weil

Whitman wrote two books about the American Civil War. His major prose work is a war-time autobiography that began as a series of six sketches published in the New York *Weekly Graphic* as ''Tis But Ten Years Since' (1874). Whitman collected and republished the *Weekly Graphic* articles as a privately printed book, *Memoranda During the War* (1875), and later incorporated most of that work into *Specimen Days and Collect* (1882). Whitman's Civil War poetry was published as *Drum-Taps* in April 1865, then re-published several months later with *Sequel to Drum-Taps* (to include his elegies on the death of Lincoln), and eventually incorporated into *Leaves of Grass* as a cluster of forty-three poems. Whitman's phrase 'Drum-Taps' combines two different sets of associations, both important for understanding his response to the war: a call to arms signaled by the percussive intensity of beating drums, and a call to reflection and mourning signaled by the bugle song, 'Taps', played at the conclusion of a military funeral. It's a good title. *Drum-Taps* begins with an unashamed celebration of what the poet calls 'ruthless force,' a militaristic drum beat that sweeps aside hesitation and compromise, the political legacy of the 1850s, and lets slip the dogs of war: 'Through the windows – through doors – burst like a ruthless force,' Whitman writes in 'Beat! Beat! Drums!' – one of his first Civil War poems:

> Make no parley – stop for no expostulation,
> Mind not the timid – mind not the weeper or prayer,

Mind not the old man beseeching the young man,
Let not the child's voice be heard.

This doesn't sound much like Walt Whitman – at least not the great tender mother-man who shares the misery of mashed firemen and hounded slaves and announces himself as Ralph Waldo Emerson's doctor-poet, raising the despairing with 'resistless will,' as he said in 'Song of Myself,' dilating them with 'tremendous breath.' In the early stage of his career Whitman celebrated the central role of the arts in American public life and argued that the proof of a poet is that his country absorbs him as surely as he absorbs it. It became abundantly clear to everyone, Whitman especially, that America had no interest in absorbing *Leaves of Grass*. The first three editions languished unsold at his publishers. And the few critics who bothered to read the book were mostly baffled or offended. (One suggested that Whitman should do the country a favor and put a bullet in his own head.) In spite of Emerson's extravagant prediction 'I greet you at the beginning of a great career,' Whitman's literary career had stalled by 1860 in a mud-thick depression he called his New York Slough. He'd lost his job as editor of the *Brooklyn Daily Times*, got his heart broken in a love affair with Fred Vaughn, and watched helplessly as his family slid further into poverty and squalor. And so he spent most days trying out a different role for himself at Pfaff's beer cellar in Greenwich Village; not Emerson's healer-poet but a wine-tippling bohemian *artiste* fending off the advances of various New York actresses and mired in a kind of world-weary malaise.

In the first edition of *Leaves of Grass* Whitman had welcomed the resurgent energies of an America freed from just that sort of hipster weariness – a broad-shouldered, big-hearted American adolescent living large in the glorious energies of this new day. 'I sound my barbaric yawp over the roofs of the world,' Whitman declared at the end of 'Song of Myself,' which is not a call to arms but a call to spiritual renewal, a revival sermon preached from the roof-tops that ends with an altar call of democratic commitment: the doors of the church are open, as American evangelists say. Preaching that sermon in full voice in 1855, Whitman invites presidents and prostitutes, stage drivers and steamship captains to sit down together at the table of mutual fellowship, what Martin Luther King Jr. called the beloved community, in a shared commitment to the dignity and goodness of common people.

That vision didn't last long. Many things changed for Whitman after the first edition of *Leaves of Grass*, but what bothered him most was the presidential election of 1856, which somehow managed to bring together the worst possible candidates for American leadership – James Buchanan, Millard Fillmore, and John C. Fremont – at the worst possible moment in American history. Things were unraveling fast. And it's difficult to understand *Drum-Taps* and *Memoranda During the War* without gauging the depth of Whitman's political disillusionment in the years leading up to the war. In an escalating series of bare-knuckle jeremiads like 'The Eighteenth Presidency!' and the poem 'Respondez!', Whitman laments the betrayal of democratic community by a rogues' gallery of political hacks.

None of this had much to do with slavery for Whitman. Those losses didn't register with anywhere near the impact of the subjugation of white working people on both sides of the Mason–Dixon line. But thinking about the lives of pennies-a-day teamsters, mechanics, and carpenters brought Whitman's blood to a boil and thickened that New York Slough. Surveying the state of the nation just before the Civil War, Whitman could see no evidence of political dignity, moral leadership, or the loving regard for others he called, with a slightly Marxist flair, *comradeship* (and which knew in his heart was the only hope of real union in a genuinely pluralistic society). None of that – and instead a gathering swarm of dandies, pimps, malignants, office-vermin, mail-riflers, and limber-tongued lawyers. What Whitman believed *he* needed, languishing in that New York bar, and what he believed *America* needed, having sold its birthright to the limber-tongued lawyers, turned out to be pretty much the same thing (as was usually the case with Whitman): a refiner's fire of cleansing violence straight out of the Old Testament, something ruthless and definitive. And so: 'Through the windows – through doors – burst like a ruthless force,/ Into the solemn church, and scatter the congregation,' as he said in 'Beat! Beat! Drums!'

That stance changed quickly. Whitman's younger brother George was wounded at the Battle of Fredericksburg on December 13, 1862, a two-day massacre of colossal proportions that gave anyone who was paying attention a clear sign that this war would have nothing to do with Napoleonic gallantry and everything to do with butchery and bloodshed – brought on by a perfect storm of political blundering, military mismanagement, and a .58-caliber rifled musket shot named, after its French inventor, the Minié bullet. There was nothing minimal about that bullet. It could be fired with accuracy from a range of over a thousand yards, and the bullet's low muzzle velocity and heavy weight meant that it was perfectly designed to produce horrific wounding. One theme in the history of Civil War medicine is the story of military surgeons performing amputations under extreme conditions with little or no knowledge of antisepsis. Seventy-one percent of Civil War wounds were to the arms, legs, hands, or feet. And the bone-crushing force of the Minié bullet meant that the only medical response in most cases was amputation, a truth brought home vividly to Whitman a few hours after he arrived in Virginia to look for his brother.

It was a nightmare journey – which got worse after Whitman arrived. George's name (misspelled as G.W. Whitmore) had appeared in the casualty reports of the *New York Tribune* on December 16, 1862. When Whitman read the paper with his family in Brooklyn, he immediately gathered his clothes and notebooks, accepted fifty dollars from his mother, and caught a train to Virginia that would change his life. It turns out that George was alive and well after the twenty-seven hour battle. His cheek was gashed by a shell fragment and his regiment was decimated by General Ambrose Burnside's catastrophic decision to order a frontal assault on the entrenched Confederate position on Marye's Heights. It was one of the worst defeats of the Union army in the entire Civil War. But George would live to fight another day. Many days, in fact. George Whitman survived twenty-one major battles, including Antietam, Cedar Mountain, Second Manassas, Chantilly, and the Battle of the Wilderness. And much of what Whitman learned about the life and suffering of Union soldiers he learned from George, 'just the luckiest man in the American army,' as one of George's comrades told Whitman.

Others weren't so lucky. One of the first things Whitman saw in Virginia was an impromptu military hospital, the Lacy mansion, where Union surgeons had created a large 'heap of feet, legs, arms, and human fragments, cut, bloody, black and blue, swelled and sickening,' as Whitman wrote in his notebook. Clara Barton, the future founder of the American Red Cross and a volunteer nurse whose personality and Civil War career almost perfectly mirrored Whitman's, happened to be present at the mansion when the poet arrived. But Whitman didn't enter the Lacy House or notice Barton working inside. Instead, his attention was drawn to the pile of amputations and a nearby row of dead bodies covered by a brown woolen blanket. Except that they didn't look like 'dead bodies' to Whitman but something more brutal and formless than that, not a human person but 'a shapeless extended object,' as he wrote in his notebook.

This is what 'ruthless force' looks like up close. War depersonalizes and dehumanizes people, as Simone Weil argues in an essay written in 1939. The true hero and subject of war is *force*, she says in her famous essay on *The Iliad*, 'that x that turns anybody who is subjected to it into a *thing*.' War is a technology of strict erasure for Weil, a Medusa-machine that turns living flesh into cold stone:

Somebody was here, and the next minute there is nobody here at all. [...] Such is the nature of force. Its power of converting a man into a thing is a double one, and in its application double-edged. To the same degree, though in different fashions, those who use it and those who endure it are turned to stone. [...] The art of war is simply the art of producing such transformations.

This is exactly what Whitman saw on that hillside in Virginia: human beings turned into shapeless objects, heroes transformed into things. And it became clear to Whitman even then that responding to such dehumanizing force would require a different sort of writing, not the barbaric yawper preaching from roof-tops but the compassionate witness or 'wound dresser' turning to face the dying and the dead.

If there's a bottom-line ethics in Whitman war writings, this is probably it: turning out to face the *other*. Whitman was interested in half a dozen visual aesthetics in this period. He was fascinated by the new science of photography and writes Civil War poems and prose sketches that resemble a Mathew Brady daguerreotype. He was intrigued by the possibilities of the literary romance, as I've argued elsewhere, and adapts techniques from Hawthorne and Poe to express what he termed in his notebook 'the romance of surgery & medicine.' He learned to blend the factual authority of direct observation (gleaned from soldiers' stories he heard in the hospital wards) with the stylistic resources of prose fiction to create a nineteenth-century version of New Journalism, as in his description of the Battle of Chancellorsville in *Memoranda During the War*, 'A Night Battle, Over a Week Since.' And Whitman explores an equally diverse range of ethical responses to the suffering of the war: the Good Death tradition of the bedside vigil (as Drew Gilpin Faust has shown), Christian traditions of redemptive suffering, and transcendental traditions of natural resurrection and pastoral healing.

But most of all, Whitman explored an ethics of intimate attention. What haunted Whitman's imagination during the war was the anonymity and abandonment of soldiers suffering or dying alone – 'untended lying,' as he said in the poem he would write about the Lacy House experience, 'A Sight in Camp in the Daybreak Gray and Dim.' Tending the dying and the dead, gazing into their faces, individualizing them in his hospital notebooks and journalism – all this became a kind of mission for Whitman, a sacred calling. After Fredericksburg, Whitman spent the next four years working part-time in the Army Paymaster's office in Washington and living with his friend and poetic champion, William O'Connor. But Whitman's real work began in the late afternoons and evenings when he would don fresh clothes, pack a knapsack with gifts of money, clothing, and food, and visit the wounded and dying soldiers in the chaotic wards of Washington hospitals: the Armory Square, the Judiciary Square, the Patent Office, and many others. Whitman estimated that he made over six hundred hospital visits during the Civil War and cared for nearly one hundred thousand soldiers from both armies – standing vigil at their bedsides, writing letters to their loved ones, fanning them during the horrific summer heat, reading aloud from Shakespeare, Sir Walter Scott, Miles O'Reilly, and the Bible (but never his own poetry). Like Mary Ann Bickerdyke and Clara Barton, Whitman worked outside of any agency or institution and saw himself as an advocate for the common soldier. His heroes are not Ulysses S. Grant or Robert E. Lee but Erastus Haskell, Lewy Brown, Thomas Sawyer, Frank Irwin, and Oscar Wilber – rank-and-file soldiers whose courage and compassion restored Whitman's faith in American democracy but whose stories remained 'untended' by traditional histories of the war.

One way Whitman cares for these soldiers is to bear witness to their lives. 'J.T.L, of company F., 9th New Hampshire, lies in bed 37, ward I. Is very fond of tobacco,' he writes in a typical passage from *Memoranda During the War.* 'Bed 3, ward E, Armory, has a great hankering for pickles, something pungent.' 'D.S.G., bed 52, wants a good book; has a sore weak throat; would like some horehound candy.' Such references to food, tobacco and books recover fragile subjectivities of appetite, inclination, heritage, and social class. They advertise exactly the kind of modest, distinguishing details that restore a sense of humanness to people in danger of falling out of the world. If one effect of ruthless force is dehumanizing erasure, as Weil argues, then the cultural work of nursing may be, in part, to reconnect badly damaged people to everyday things and routines: the remembered taste of a certain kind of food, for instance, or the individualizing pleasure of a particular book.

But that sort of response requires a unique quality of attention. Much is made of the totalizing tendency in Whitman's writing, his use of universals and long shots to absorb particularizing difference in a wide-angle Emersonian gaze. What Whitman stresses in his hospital writings is nearly the opposite of that: a way of seeing that notices and cherishes individual faces and needs, right down to the horehound candy. This kind of response turns the nurse or wound dresser out of himself. It interrupts an ego-centered subject secure in his own skin or steady in his own stance and sets the moral focus just beyond the nucleus of the private self, displacing attention from center to edge, self to other. This is the basic grammar of poetry and metaphor, of course – *trope* means turn. But this is also the basic grammar of moral attention for Whitman, the sign of a person inflected by the needs of other people and turning toward them in sympathetic response: bending down to the faces of children ('The Wound-Dresser'); stepping aside to see the faces of the dead ('A Sight in Camp in the Daybreak Gray and Dim'); breaking ranks to hold vigil for a fallen comrade ('Vigil Strange I Kept on the Field One Night'); looking up to meet the gaze of suffering patients, as in this scene from Whitman's Civil War journalism: 'Reader, how can I describe to you the mute appealing look that rolls and moves from many a manly eye, from many a sick cot, following you as you walk slowly down one of these wards?' ('The Great Army of the Sick').

That rolling look followed Whitman everywhere, even in his sleep. Responding to its mute appeal inscribes an ethics of uncertain balance and precarious turning for Whitman, what the French philosopher and Holocaust survivor Emmanuel Levinas calls the 'moral summons' of the face (*Totality and Infinity*). This sort of moral stance fits a person who's not all that self-reliant or self-composed, the goal of much of Whitman's writing before the war, but suggests instead a subject continually interrupted by the impinging presence of other people and so vigilant and hyper-alert: a 'sleepless' witness in Whitman ('A Sight in Camp'); a moral 'insomniac' in Levinas (*Entre-Nous: Thinking of the Other*).

To express this moral vigilance, Whitman adopts a different rhythm in his war writings – not the straight-line plot of traditional narrative but the dilatory pace of hesitating, pausing, stepping aside. Living this way felt deeply religious to Whitman but religion without church or creed, a moral philosophy for beginners, as Levinas would say, where what matters isn't fixed faith or unswerving belief but a capacity for small acts of sacred attention: bending down to the face of the other, turning out toward that rolling eye. And so Whitman privileges scenes of partial recognition in his war writings, the glance from across the room he'd perfected in the *Calamus* poems, but more fragile and uncertain than that: eyes opening from sleep or anesthesia and then closing again; a stranger materializing from out of a crowd or in the midst of a parade and then disappearing; faces glimpsed through smoke or tears; faces emerging from behind a hospital curtain; faces revealed by candlelight or campfire; flickering faces visible and then gone. The memory of those faces would haunt Whitman for the rest of his life and call out from him some of the most beautiful writing of his career. Not the drum beats of militaristic force but psalms of elegy and quiet lament, the bugle song at close of day.

References

Davis, Robert Leigh, *Whitman and the Romance of Medicine* (Berkeley: University of California Press, 1997).

Faust, Drew Gilpin, *This Republic of Suffering: Death and the American Civil War* (New York: Vintage, 2008).

Levinas, Emmanuel, *Entre-Nous: Thinking of the Other*, Trans. Michael B. Smith and Barbara Harshav (New York: Columbia University Press, 1998).

——, *Totality and Infinity: An Essay on Exteriority*, Trans. Alphonso Lingis (Pittsburgh: Duquesne University Press, 1969).

Weil, Simone, 'The *Iliad* or the Poem of Force,' in *Simone Weil: An Anthology*, ed. Siân Miles (New York: Grove Press, 1986), pp. 162–95.

Whitman, Walt, *Notebooks and Unpublished Prose Manuscripts*, Vol. 2, ed. Edward F. Grier (New York: New York University Press, 1984).

——, 'The Great Army of the Sick,' *New York Times*, February 26, 1863, reprinted in Richard M. Bucke, ed., *The Wound Dresser: A Series of Letters Written in Washington During the War of Rebellion* (Boston: Small, Maynard, 1898), pp. 5–6.

——, *Walt Whitman: Complete Poetry and Collected Prose*, ed. Justin Kaplan (New York: Literary Classics of the United States, 1982).

——, *Walt Whitman's 'Memoranda During the War' and Death of Abraham Lincoln*, ed. Roy P. Basler (Bloomington: Indiana University Press, 1962).

Specimen Days & Collect

Walt Whitman (1819–1892) became actively involved in the Civil War in 1862 when he heard that his brother, George Washington Whitman, had been wounded in the Battle of Fredericksburg. Though the injury was only superficial, Whitman stayed on in Washington, visiting the Armory Square Hospital, among others, and tending to the wounded with a missionary zeal. 'Down at the Front' was Whitman's only first-hand account of battle and became the basis of his poem 'A Sight in Camp in the Daybreak Gray and Dim' (included in *Drum-Taps*). 'A Night Battle' pieces together soldiers' accounts of the Battle of Chancellorsville and exemplifies Whitman's method of description through cumulative visual detail. 'Some Specimen Cases' is, as the title suggests, a series of case notes. 'The Real War Will Never Get in the Books' expresses his scepticism about the depiction of the Civil War, which was already by the mid-1860s emerging as a major cultural issue.

Texts taken from Walt Whitman, *Specimen Days & Collect* (Philadelphia: Rees Welch, 1882). The text of *Memoranda during the War* (Camden, NJ: author's publication, 1875–76) can be found at http://web.archive.org/web/20080718102114/http://etext.lib. virginia.edu/toc/modeng/public/WhiMemo.html. See also Peter Coviello, ed., *Walt Whitman's Memoranda during the War* (New York: Oxford University Press, 2004).

DOWN AT THE FRONT

[Lacy House] FALMOUTH, VA., *opposite Fredericksburgh, December 21, 1862.* – Begin my visits among the camp hospitals in the army of the Potomac. Spend a good part of the day in a large brick mansion on the banks of the Rappahannock, used as a hospital since the battle – seems to have receiv'd only the worst cases. Out doors, at the foot of a tree, within ten yards of the front of the house, I notice a heap of amputated feet, legs, arms, hands, &c., a full load for a one-horse cart. Several dead bodies lie near, each cover'd with its brown woolen blanket. In the door-yard, towards the river, are fresh graves, mostly of officers, their names on pieces of barrel-staves or broken boards, stuck in the dirt. (Most of these bodies were subsequently taken up and transported north to their friends.) The large mansion is quite crowded upstairs and down, everything impromptu, no system, all bad enough, but I have no doubt the best that can be done; all the wounds pretty bad, some frightful, the men in their old clothes, unclean and bloody. Some of the wounded are rebel soldiers and officers, prisoners. One, a Mississippian, a captain, hit badly in leg, I talk'd with some time; he ask'd me for papers, which I gave him. (I saw him three months afterward in Washington, with his leg amputated, doing well.) I went through the rooms, downstairs and up. Some of the men were dying. I had nothing to give at that visit, but wrote a few letters to folks home, mothers, &c. Also talk'd to three or four, who seem'd most susceptible to it, and needing it.

A NIGHT BATTLE OVER A WEEK SINCE

May 12. – There was part of the late battle at Chancellorsville, (second Fredericksburgh,) a little over a week ago, Saturday, Saturday night and Sunday, under Gen. Joe Hooker, I would like to give just a glimpse of – (a moment's look in a terrible storm at sea – of which a few suggestions are enough, and full details impossible.) The fighting had been very hot during the day, and after an intermission the latter part, was resumed at night, and kept up with furious energy till 3 o'clock in the morning. That afternoon (Saturday) an attack sudden and strong by Stonewall Jackson had gain'd a great advantage to the southern army, and broken our lines, entering us like a wedge, and leaving things in that position at dark. But Hooker at 11 at night made a desperate push, drove the secesh [secessionist] forces back, restored his original lines, and resumed his plans. This night scrimmage was very exciting, and afforded countless strange and fearful pictures. The fighting had been general both at Chancellorsville and northeast at Fredericksburgh. (We hear of some poor fighting, episodes, skedaddling on our part. I think not of it. I think of the fierce bravery, the general rule.) One corps, the 6th, Sedgewick's, fights four dashing and bloody battles in thirty-six hours, retreating in great jeopardy, losing largely but maintaining itself, fighting with the sternest desperation under all circumstances, getting over the Rappahannock only by the skin of its teeth, yet getting over. It lost many, many brave men, yet it took vengeance, ample vengeance.

But it was the tug of Saturday evening, and through the night and Sunday morning, I wanted to make a special note of. It was largely in the woods, and quite a general engagement. The night was very pleasant, at times the moon shining out full and clear, all Nature so calm in itself, the early summer grass so rich, and foliage of the trees – yet there the battle raging, and many good fellows lying helpless, with new accessions to them, and every minute amid the rattle of muskets and crash of cannon, (for there was an artillery contest too,) the red life-blood oozing out from heads or trunks or limbs upon that green and dew-cool grass. Patches of the woods take fire, and several of the wounded, unable to move, are consumed – quite large spaces are swept over, burning the dead also – some of the men have their hair and beards singed – some, burns on their faces and hands – others holes burnt in their clothing. The flashes of fire from the cannon, the quick flaring flames and smoke, and the immense roar – the musketry so general, the light nearly bright enough for each side to see the other – the crashing, tramping of men – the yelling – close quarters – we hear the secesh yells – our men cheer loudly back, especially if Hooker is in sight – hand to hand conflicts, each side stands up to it, brave, determin'd as demons, they often charge upon us – a thousand deeds are done worth to write newer greater poems on – and still the woods on fire – still many are not only scorch'd – too many, unable to move, are burned to death.

Then the camps of the wounded – O heavens, what scene is this? – is this indeed *humanity* – these butchers' shambles? There are several of them. There they lie, in the largest, in an open space in the woods, from 200 to 300 poor fellows – the groans and screams – the odor of blood, mixed with the fresh scent of the night, the grass, the trees – that slaughter-house! O well is it their mothers, their sisters cannot see them – cannot conceive, and never conceiv'd, these things. One man is shot by a shell, both in the arm and leg – both are amputated – there lie the rejected members. Some have their legs blown off – some bullets through the breast – some indescribably horrid wounds in the face or head, all mutilated, sickening, torn, gouged out – some in the abdomen – some mere boys – many rebels, badly hurt – they take their regular turns with the rest, just the same as any – the surgeons use them just the same. Such is the camp of the wounded – such a fragment, a reflection afar off of the bloody scene – while all over the clear, large moon comes out at times softly, quietly shining. Amid the woods, that scene of flitting souls – amid the crack and crash and yelling sounds – the impalpable perfume of the woods – and yet the pungent, stifling smoke – the radiance of the moon, looking from heaven at intervals so placid – the sky so heavenly the clear-obscure up there, those buoyant upper oceans – a few large placid stars beyond, coming silently and languidly out, and then disappearing – the melancholy, draperied night above, around. And there, upon the roads, the fields, and in those woods, that contest, never one more desperate in any age or land – both parties now in force – masses – no fancy battle, no semi-play, but fierce and savage demons fighting there – courage and scorn of death the rule, exceptions almost none.

SOME SPECIMEN CASES

June 18th. – In one of the hospitals I find Thomas Haley, company M, 4th New York cavalry – a regular Irish boy, a fine specimen of youthful physical manliness – shot through the lungs – inevitably dying – came over to this country from Ireland to enlist – has not a single friend or acquaintance here – is sleeping soundly at this moment, (but it is the sleep of death) – has a bullet-hole straight through the lung. I saw Tom when first brought here, three days since, and didn't suppose he could live twelve hours – (yet he looks well enough in the face to a casual observer.) He lies there with his frame exposed above the waist, all naked, for coolness, a fine built man, the tan not yet bleach'd from his cheeks and neck. It is useless to talk to him, as with his sad hurt, and the stimulants they give him, and the utter strangeness of every object, face, furniture, &c., the poor fellow, even when awake, is like some frighten'd, shy animal. Much of the time he sleeps, or half sleeps. (Sometimes I thought he knew more than he show'd.) I often come and sit by him in perfect silence; he will breathe for ten minutes as softly and evenly as a young babe asleep. Poor youth, so handsome, athletic, with profuse beautiful shining hair. One time as I sat looking at him while he lay asleep, he suddenly, without the least start, awaken'd, open'd his eyes, gave me a long steady look, turning his face very slightly to gaze easier – one long, clear, silent look – a slight sigh – then turn'd back and went into his doze again. Little he knew, poor death-stricken boy, the heart of the stranger that hover'd near.

W.H.E., Co. F, 2nd N.Y. – His disease is pneumonia. He lay sick at the wretched hospital below Aquia creek, for seven or eight days before brought here. He was detail'd from his regiment to go there and help as nurse, but was soon taken down himself. Is an elderly, sallow-faced, rather gaunt, gray-hair'd man, a widower, with children. He express'd a great desire for good, strong green tea. An excellent lady, Mrs. W., of Washington, soon sent him a package; also a small sum of money. The doctor said give him the tea at pleasure; it lay on the table by his side, and he used it every day. He slept a great deal; could not talk much, as he grew deaf. Occupied bed 15, ward I, Armory. (The same lady above, Mrs. W., sent the men a large package of tobacco.)

J.G. lies in bed 52, ward I; is of company B, 7th Pennsylvania. I gave him a small sum of money, some tobacco, and envelopes. To a man adjoining also gave twenty-five cents; he flush'd in the face when I offer'd it – refused at first, but as I found he had not a cent, and was very fond of having the daily papers to read, I prest it on him. He was evidently very grateful, but said little.

J.T.L., of company F, 9th New Hampshire, lies in bed 37, ward I. Is very fond of tobacco. I furnish him some; also with a little money. Has gangrene of the feet; a pretty bad case; will surely have to lose three toes. Is a regular specimen of an old-fashion'd, rude, hearty, New England countryman, impressing me with his likeness to that celebrated singed cat, who was better than she look'd.

Bed 3, ward E, Armory, has a great hankering for pickles, something pungent. After consulting the doctor, I gave him a small bottle of horse-radish; also some apples; also a book. Some of the nurses are excellent. The woman-nurse in this ward I like very much. (Mrs. Wright – a year afterwards I found her in Mansion house hospital, Alexandria – she is a perfect nurse.)

In one bed a young man, Marcus Small, company K, 7th Maine – sick with dysentery and typhoid fever – pretty critical case – I talk with him often – he thinks he will die – looks like it indeed. I write a letter for him home to East Livermore, Maine – I let him talk to me a little, but not much, advise him to keep very quiet – do most of the talking myself – stay quite a while with him, as he holds on to my hand – talk to him in a cheering, but slow, low and measured manner – talk about his furlough, and going home as soon as he is able to travel.

Thomas Lindly, 1st Pennsylvania cavalry, shot very badly through the foot – poor young man, he suffers horridly, has to be constantly dosed with morphine, his face ashy and glazed, bright young eyes – I give him a large handsome apple, lay it in sight, tell him to have it roasted in the morning, as he generally feels easier then, and can eat a little breakfast. I write two letters for him.

Opposite, an old Quaker lady sits by the side of her son, Amer Moore, 2d U.S. artillery – shot in the head two weeks since, very low, quite rational – from hips down paralyzed – he will surely die. I speak a very few words to him every day and evening – he answers pleasantly – wants nothing – (he told me soon after he came about his home affairs, his mother had been an invalid, and he fear'd to let her know his condition.) He died soon after she came.

THE REAL WAR WILL NEVER GET IN THE BOOKS

And so good-bye to the war. I know not how it may have been, or may be, to others – to me the main interest I found, (and still, on recollection, find,) in the rank and file of the armies, both sides, and in those specimens amid the hospitals, and even the dead on the field. To me the points illustrating the latent personal character and eligibilities of these States, in the two or three millions of American young and middle-aged men, North and South, embodied in those armies – and especially the one-third or one-fourth of their number, stricken by wounds or disease at some time in the course of the contest – were of more significance even than the political interests involved. (As so much of a race depends on how it faces death, and how it stands personal anguish and sickness. As, in the glints of emotions under emergencies, and the indirect traits and asides in Plutarch, we get far profounder clues to the antique world than all its more formal history.)

Future years will never know the seething hell and the black infernal background of countless minor scenes and interiors, (not the official surface-courteousness of the Generals, not the few great battles) of the Secession war; and it is best they should not – the real war will never get in the books. In the mushy influences of current times, too, the fervid atmosphere and typical events of those years are in danger of being totally forgotten. I have at night watch'd by the side of a sick man in the hospital, one who could not live many hours. I have seen his eyes flash and burn as he raised himself and recurr'd to the cruelties on his surrender'd brother, and mutilations of the corpse afterward. (See in the preceding pages, the incident at Upperville – the seventeen kill'd as in the description, were left there on the ground. After they dropt dead, no one touch'd them – all were made sure of, however. The carcasses were left for the citizens to bury or not, as they chose.)

Such was the war. It was not a quadrille in a ball-room. Its interior history will not only never be written – its practicality, minutia; of deeds and passions, will never be even suggested. The actual soldier of 1862-'65, North and South, with all his ways, his incredible dauntlessness, habits, practices, tastes, language, his fierce friendship, his appetite, rankness, his superb strength and animality, lawless gait, and a hundred unnamed lights and shades of camp, I say, will never be written – perhaps must not and should not be.

The preceding notes may furnish a few stray glimpses into that life, and into those lurid interiors, never to be fully convey'd to the future. The hospital part of the drama from '61 to '65, deserves indeed to be recorded. Of that many-threaded drama, with its sudden and strange surprises, its confounding of prophecies, its moments of despair, the dread of foreign interference, the interminable campaigns, the bloody battles, the mighty and cumbrous and green armies, the drafts and bounties – the immense money expenditure, like a heavy-pouring constant rain – with, over the whole land, the last three years of the struggle, an unending, universal mourning-wail of women, parents, orphans – the marrow of the tragedy concentrated in those Army Hospitals – (it seem'd sometimes as if the whole interest of the land, North and South, was one vast central hospital, and all the rest of the affair but flanges) – those forming the untold and unwritten history of the war – infinitely greater (like life's) than the few scraps and distortions that are ever told or written. Think how much, and of importance, will be – how much, civic and military, has already been – buried in the grave, in eternal darkness.

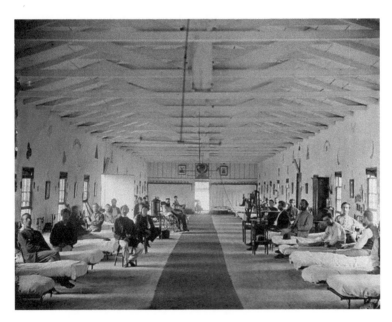

Figure 3: Armory Square Hospital, Washington, DC

MEDICAL FACILITIES AND PATHOLOGY

Jonathan Letterman
on the Medical Corps

Jonathan Letterman (1824–1872) was a surgeon who in 1862 was appointed Medical Director of the Army of the Potomac. He revolutionized medical care in the battlefield by introducing a holistic system of fresh supplies, evacuation practice and mobile hospitals, including medical provision for the thousands of wounded after the Battle of Gettysburg. The following excerpt is taken from Jonathan Letterman, *Medical Recollections of the Army of the Potomac* (New York: Appleton, 1866). For further details, see Bennett A. Clements, 'Memoir of Jonathan Letterman,' *Journal of the Military Service Institution* 4, No. 15 (September 1888).

I am convinced that there exists in the minds of many, perhaps the majority, of line officers, a very imperfect conception of the position of Medical officers, and the objects for which a Medical Staff was instigated. It is a popular delusion that the highest duties of Medical officers are performed in prescribing a drug or amputating a limb; and the troops frequently feel the ill effect of this obsolete idea, and are often unnecessarily broken down in health and compelled to endure suffering which would have been avoided did commanders take a comprehensive view of this important subject. It is a matter of surprise that such a prejudice should exist in this enlightened age, particularly among highly intelligent men; and it were well if commanding officers would disabuse their minds of it, and permit our armies to profit more fully by the beneficial advice of those who, for years, have made the laws of life a study, and who are therefore best able to counteract the influences which so constantly tend to undermine the health of the army and destroy its efficiency. A corps of Medical officers was not established solely for the purpose of attending the wounded and sick; the proper treatment of these sufferers is certainly a matter of very great importance, and is an imperative duty, but the labours of Medical officers cover a more extended field. The leading idea, which should be constantly in view, is to strengthen the hands of the Commanding General by keeping his army in the most vigorous health, thus rendering it in the highest degree, efficient for enduring fatigue and privation, and for fighting.

The Confederate Military Prison Hospital
at Andersonville, Georgia

Austin Flint (1812–1886) was an American Physician who pioneered the study of heart disease. He held a chair in clinical medicine in New Orleans before moving to New York. From 1861 to 1868 he served as professor of pathology in Long Island College Hospital. The following excerpt is taken from Chapter 3 of Austin Flint, ed., *Contributions Relating to the Causes and Prevention of Disease, and to Camp Diseases; Together with a Report a Report of the Diseases, etc. among the Prisoners at Andersonville, Ga.* (New York: Hurd and Houghton, 1867). Published for the US Sanitary Commission.

The US Sanitary Commission was established in 1861, with its headquarters in Washington, DC, to support Union casualties. From 1863 its members organized fund-raising Sanitary Fairs. The Commission established hospitals and rest homes, continuing operation after the war. The official account of its activities is Charles J. Stille's *History of the United States Sanitary Commission, Being the General Report of Its Work during the War of the Rebellion* (Philadelphia: J.B. Lippincott, 1866), at https://archive.org/details/historyofuniteds00stiluoft.

The preface announces that the Commission 'has not hesitated to criticize with the utmost freedom the policy and measures of the Government, where they seemed radically defective in providing for the care and comfort of the sick and suffering of the Army' (v–vi).

The Hospital is situated near the southeastern corner situation of the Stockade, and covers about five acres of ground.

The larger forest trees, as the pine and oak, have been left in their natural state, and furnish pleasant shade to the patients.

The ground slopes gently toward the south arid east. A sluggish stream of water flows through the southern portion of the hospital grounds from west to east. The upper portion of this stream is used by the patients for washing their clothes, whilst along the borders of the lower portions logs have been ranged upon which the patients may sit and evacuate their bowels. This part of the stream was a semi-fluid mass of human excrements, offal, and filth of all kinds.

This immense cesspool, fermenting beneath the hot sun, emitted an overpowering stench.

The banks of this stream south of the hospital inclosure [sic] are bordered by a swamp which spreads out toward the southeast. This swamp is well covered by forest trees, usual in southern swamps, as the small magnolia, red bay, sweet gums, black gum, tupelo, tulip-tree, red maple, ash, and beech.

North of the hospital grounds, the stream which flows through the Stockade pursues its sluggish and filthy course. The exhalations from this swamp, which is loaded with the excrements of the prisoners confined in the Stockade, exert their deleterious influences upon the inmates of the Hospital.

The entire grounds are surrounded by a frail board fence, and are strictly guarded by Confederate soldiers, and no prisoner, except the paroled attendants, is allowed to leave the grounds except by a special permit from the commandant of the interior of the prison.

The patients and attendants, near two thousand in number, are crowded into this confined space, and are but poorly supplied with old and ragged tents. Large numbers of them were without any bunks, and lay upon the ground, ofttimes without even a blanket – no beds or straw appear to have been furnished.

The tents extend to within a few yards of the small stream, the eastern portion of which, as we have before said, was used as a privy, and was loaded with excrements; and I observed a large pile of corn-bread, bones, and filth of all kinds, thirty feet in diameter and several feet in height, swarming with myriads of flies, in a vacant space near the pots used for cooking.

Millions of flies swarmed over everything, and covered the faces of the sleeping patients, and crawled down their open mouths and deposited their maggots in the gangrenous wounds of the living and in the mouths of the dead. Myriads of mosquitoes also infested the tents, and many of the patients were so stung by these pestiferous insects that they appeared as if they were suffering from a slight attack of measles.

The police and hygiene of the hospital was defective in the extreme; as the attendants were selected from the prisoners, they not only robbed the sick of their clothing and rations, but also neglected their comfort and cleanliness in a most shameful manner. The sick were literally incrusted with dirt and covered with vermin.

When a gangrenous wound needed washing, the limb was thrust out a little from the blanket or board or rags upon which the patient was lying, and water poured over it, and all the putrescent matters allowed to soak into the ground floor of the tent.

The supply of rags for dressing wounds was said to be very scant; and I saw the most filthy rags, which had been applied several times and imperfectly washed, used in dressing recent wounds. When hospital gangrene was prevailing it was impossible for any wound to escape contagion under these circumstances.

I saw several gangrenous wounds filled with maggots. The numerous flies which swarmed around and over every ulcer, without doubt formed efficient agents for the spread of hospital gangrene.

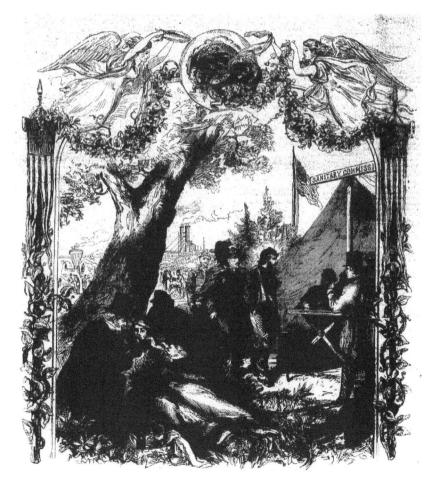

Figure 4: The Sanitary Commission

Field Hospitals: A Glimpse

John B. Billings (1842–?) served in the 10th Massachusetts Battery of Light Artillery, and after the war published *Hardtack and Coffee or, The Unwritten Story of Army Life* (Boston, MA: George H. Smith, 1887). The memoir was illustrated by pen and ink drawings by Charles W. Reed, a topographical engineer on General Warren's staff.

I vividly remember my first look into one of these field hospitals. It was, I think, on the 27th of November, 1863, during the Mine Run Campaign, so-called. General French, then commanding the Third Corps, was fighting the battle of Locust Grove, and General Warren, with the Second Corps, had also been engaged with the enemy, and had driven him from the neighbourhood of Robertson's Tavern, in the vicinity of which the terrific Battle of the Wilderness began the following May. Near this tavern the field hospital of Warren's Second Division had been located, and into this I peered while my battery stood in park not far away, awaiting orders. The surgeon had just completed an operation. It was the amputation of an arm about five inches below the shoulder, the stump being now carefully dressed and bandaged. As soon as the patient recovered from the effects of the ether, the attendants raised him to a sitting posture on the operating-table. At that moment the thought of his wounded arm returned to him, and, turning his eyes towards it, they met only the projecting stub. The awful reality dawned upon him for the first time. An arm had gone forever, and he dropped backwards on the table in a swoon. Many a poor fellow like him brought to the operator's table came to consciousness only to miss an arm or a leg which perhaps he had begged in his last conscious moments to have spared. But the medical officers first mentioned decided all such cases, and the patient had only to submit. At Peach-Tree Creek, Col. Thomas Reynolds of the Western army was shot in the leg, and, while the surgeons were debating the propriety of amputating it, the colonel, who was of Irish birth, begged them to spare it, as it was very valuable, being *an imported leg* – a piece of wit which saved the gallant officer his leg, although he became so much of a cripple that he was compelled to leave the service.

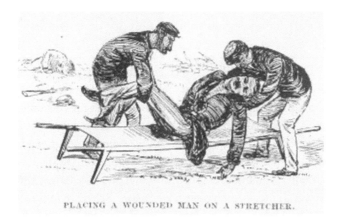

Figure 5: 'Placing a wounded man on a stretcher'
(from Billings, *Hardtack and Coffee*)

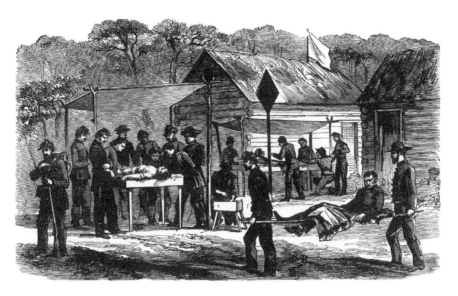

Figure 6: Field Hospital

Field Hospitals: The Need

Samuel David Gross (1805–1884) served as a surgeon in Kentucky and Philadelphia, his activities being commemorated in Thomas Eakins' painting 'The Gross Clinic.' The following text is taken from Chapter 4 ('Medical Equipments, Stores and Hospitals') of his *A Manual of Military Surgery, or Hints on the Emergencies of Field, Camp and Hospital Practice* (Philadelphia: J.B. Lippincott, 1861).

William A. Hammond (Surgeon-General of the Army, 1862–64) published *A Treatise on Hygiene with Special Reference to the Military Service* (Philadelphia: J.B. Lippincott, 1863), which specified the layout of field hospitals, stressing the prime danger of overcrowding. Hammond divides his subject into three sections: the examination of recruits, 'inherent' and external agents affecting health. He discusses a whole range of factors ranging from clean air to water filters and the role of alcohol in retarding the degeneration of tissue. In 1862 he founded the Army Medical Museum, but was dismissed from the army in 1864 on charges trumped up by the Secretary of War. After the Civil War Hammond pioneered the study of mental illness.

Besides these means, every regiment should be furnished with an ambulance, or, as the term literally implies, a movable hospital, that is, a place for the temporary accommodation and treatment of the wounded on the field of battle. It should be arranged in the form of a tent, and be provided with all the means and appliances necessary for the prompt succour of the sufferers. The materials of which it consists should be as light as possible, possess every facility for rapid packing and erection, and be conveyed from point to point by a wagon set apart for this object. The ambulance, for the invention and improvement of which we are indebted to two eminent French military surgeons, Percy and Larrey, is indispensable in every well-regulated army. This temporary hospital should be placed in an open space, convenient to water, and upon dry ground, with arrangements for the free admission of air and light, which, next to pure air, is one of the most powerful stimulants in all cases of accident attended with excessive prostration. The direct rays of the sun, in hot weather, must of course be excluded, and it may even be necessary, as in injuries of the head and eye, to wrap the patient in complete darkness. A properly regulated temperature is also to be maintained, a good average being about 68° of Fahrenheit's thermometer.

Plea for an Ambulance Service

Henry Ingersoll Bowditch (1808–1892) served as a Northern physician and published a pamphlet after his son Nathaniel died from wounds in battle: *A Brief Plea for an Ambulance System for the Army of the United States, as drawn from the extra sufferings of the late Lieut. Bowditch and a wounded comrade* (Boston: Ticknor and Fields, 1863). An ambulance corps was established in 1864.

I beg leave to state that Lieut. Bowditch, having been mortally wounded, in the first charge made after leaving Kelly's Ford, lay helpless on the ground, for some time, by the side of his dead horse. Two surgeons saw him, but they evidently had no means for carrying off the wounded officer, and it is believed *no one connected with an Ambulance Corps ever approached him there*.

A stranger horseman – probably from the Rhode Island forces – finally assisted him to get into a saddle; and he rode off, leaning over the neck of the animal – a terrible mode of proceeding, considering his severe wound in the abdomen. All this happened *when he was in the rear of our victorious army*, or, in other words, at just the place and time, at which a thorough Ambulance Corps should have been busily at work, seeking out, and relieving, with every means *a great Government should have had at its disposal*, the wretched and, perhaps, dying sufferers. But what, in reality, does the Government do to meet such an emergency? It provides a carriage, which a perfectly healthy man would find exceedingly uncomfortable to drive in, even for a few miles, and one driver, sometimes not the most humane. There are, also, I doubt not, various articles of surgical dressings, etc., for the wounded; but these articles are generally far in the rear of the army. The United States Government did not then, and never does, provide *any men*, whose duty it is to hasten to meet and to relieve these hours of poignant suffering. After Lieut. Bowditch arrived at the ambulance carriage, there was no water to be found in the casks, connected with it, although, bylaw, there should have been. The driver was wholly ignorant of the names of those whom he was carrying. He actually, and

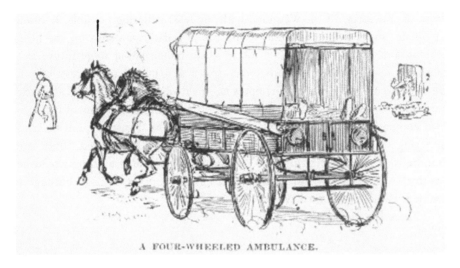

A FOUR-WHEELED AMBULANCE.

Figure 7: 'A Four-Wheeled Ambulance'
(from Billings, *Hardtack and Coffee*)

in answer to a direct question from Col. Curtis, denied that Lieut. Bowditch was one of them. He did not get any water for the Lieutenant and his still more suffering comrade, although *both longed and asked for it! A wretched and dying Sergeant begged much for it, and in vain!* Had it not been for the kindness of Col. Curtis, who, *after much difficulty*, found out where my son was, no water would probably have been procured for either of the parched sufferers. As it was, it arrived at last, *too late* for the Sergeant, who was so much exhausted as to be unable to avail himself of the cup, finally proffered him by his wounded comrade.

[...]

By having such a corps, the number of combatants would not be so rapidly lessened, as it is now, by several men taking one wounded from the field. Such an ambulance corps should consist of able-bodied, brave men – men not afraid to go to the front to save a fallen fellow-man. They should have a distinctive uniform. Arrangements might be concluded whereby the ambulance corps, in both armies, should be considered as the laws of war usually regard pickets, that is, as not to be molested in their specific duties, save perhaps, under extraordinary circumstances. Doubtless, many of such a body would fall, but it would be from random shots, and not from the voluntary barbarism of either army. It would be a brave, and noble, Christian death. Such a corps should take its place near the battle-field. It should be well trained to march, immediately to raise and carry off the wounded with the least suffering possible. It could attend to minor points of surgery, and act as nurses, or cooks on the field, in tent, and in hospital, &c. Is it too much to hope that, at some future day, similar corps, from any two belligerent armies, will, under certain restrictions, be allowed to mingle together, upon the field, more immediately after the termination of a battle, than is now allowed? If, by mutual agreement between two contending parties, this object could be gained, a vast amount of *extra* suffering would be prevented, and, doubtless, many lives saved. There are hundreds of details, that might be named, in which such a corps would be invaluable. Every great European nation has such, in its armies, thoroughly trained. Why cannot we have such?

There is no *valid* reason.

Hospital Broadside

The following is a broadside posted at the Way-Side Hospital in Salisbury, North Carolina, in 1863. The quotation in the first sentence comes from Byron's poem 'The Destruction of Sennacherib,' depicting the campaign to capture Jerusalem.

AN APPEAL

For the Sick and Wounded Soldiers.

SALISBURY, May 7th, 1863.

The brave soldiers of our Army on the Rappahannock have again met the enemy on the field of battle and scattered them 'Like leaves of the forest when autumn hath blown.' The flag of our young Republic floats gloriously over another field of blood. But victory is obtained at a fearful cost. The best blood of our nation has been shed freely on the Rappahannock, and in addition to those who have fallen in death, there are thousands of others who are wounded and disabled from present service. These will seek their own quiet homes as soon as their wounds will admit of their removal; some, whose wounds are not so serious, will come at once; others as soon as they are able. While on their way home they need places where they can obtain rest and refreshment without charge. Such a place is the Salisbury Way-Side Hospital, where more than twelve hundred of our sick and wounded soldiers have been fed and lodged, and clothed, and nursed since July last, and where all who come in the future shall be carefully provided for. But we need provisions, medicines, delicacies for the sick, and money. Will you help us now to take care of your own, or your neighbour's sons and brothers and fathers, who have so bravely fought and bled for us on the terrible fields of the Rappahannock? It is not the Hospital Committee that calls on you, it is the voice of the poor maimed and bleeding soldier that asks of you to give him 'food and fire' in exchange for the blood he has shed for you. A word to the patriotic is sufficient.

Hospitals in Richmond, Virginia

Mary Chesnut (1823–1886) was a South Carolina author married to James Chesnut, Jr., a senator and Confederate officer. She kept her diary from 1861to 1865. Gilland's was a factory converted for hospital use. The St. Charles was a former hotel, similarly converted. The following is from Chesnut's *A Diary from Dixie*, ed. Isabella D. Martin and Myrta Lockett Avary (New York: D. Appleton, 1905).

August 23 1861. Oh, such a day! Since I wrote this morning, I have been with Mrs. Randolph to all the hospitals. I can never again shut out of view the sights I saw there of human misery. I sit thinking, shut my eyes, and see it all; thinking, yes, and there is enough to think about now, God knows. Gilland's was the worst, with long rows of ill men on cots, ill of typhoid fever, of every human ailment; on dinner-tables for eating and drinking, wounds being dressed; all the horrors to be taken in at one glance.

Then we went to the St. Charles. Horrors upon horrors again; want of organization, long rows of dead and dying; awful sights. A boy from home had sent for me. He was dying in a cot, ill of fever. Next him a man died in convulsions as we stood there. I was making arrangements with a nurse, hiring him to take care of this lad; but I do not remember any more, for I fainted. Next that I knew of, the doctor and Mrs. Randolph were having me, a limp rag, put into a carriage at the door of the hospital. Fresh air, I dare say, brought me to. As we drove home the doctor came along with us, I was so upset.

Malingering

The following is from William Williams Keen, 'Surgical Reminiscences of the Civil War.' The essay referred to is William W. Keen, S. Weir Mitchell, and George W. Morehouse, 'On Malingering, especially in Regard to Simulation of Diseases of the Nervous System,' *American Journal of the Medical Sciences* 48 (October 1864), pp. 367–94. The same three authors also published *Gunshot Wounds and Other Injuries of Nerves* (Philadelphia: J.B. Lippincott, 1864).

Very naturally among so many soldiers of diverse character, and especially of men with wounds and injuries of the nervous system, we had perhaps more than our usual proportion of malingerers. In the *American Journal of the Medical Sciences* for October, 1864, p. 367, in a paper on 'Malingering,' especially in regard to simulation of diseases of the nervous system, a number of our conclusions were stated. From the necessity of the case, we devised some new means for discovering such malingerers. We first suggested the use of ether (alone or in combination with other means) as a test in a number of alleged diseases and conditions in which it had never before been used. It proved a most efficient method of detection. For instance, in asserted blindness, we suggested that the man should be etherized, the sound eye then covered with adhesive plaster, and when recovering from the anaesthetic, before he was able to reason and guard himself against making mistakes, that his sight should be tested by very simple means, such as holding out to him in the hand some water or some whiskey, or any other act which would reveal the presence or absence of sight in the supposed blind eye. So in deafness we discovered some malingerers by the old trick of gradually lowering the voice; but hearing, like sight, can best be tested during the recovery stage of ether when the patient is taken unawares, as Parr, in his 'Medical Dictionary,' speaks of a man who pretended to be dumb, of whom a sympathetic passer-by, with most insidious humanity, inquired: 'How long have you been dumb, my good friend?' 'Three weeks, sir,' replied the uncautious deceiver.

The next text is from George Cary Eggleston (1839–1911), *A Rebel's Recollections* (Cambridge, MA: The Riverside Press, 1875), Chapter 7 ('Some Queer People'). The sketches first appeared in the *Atlantic Monthly*.

Malingering became widespread in the Civil War because of the $300 bounty given recruits. The medical authorities applied anaesthetics, cauterization and the application of electrical currents to try to spot malingerers.

Among other odd specimens we had in our battery the most ingenious malingerer I ever heard of. He was in service four years, drew his pay regularly, was of robust frame and in perfect health always, and yet during the whole time he was never off the sick-list for a single day. His capacity to endure contempt was wholly unlimited, else he would have been shamed by the gibes of the men, the sneers of the surgeons, and the denunciations of the officers, into some show, at least, of a disposition to do duty. He spent the greater part of his time in hospital, never staying in camp a moment longer than he was obliged to do. When discharged, as a well man, from one hospital, he would start toward his command, and continue in that direction till he came to another infirmary, when he would have a relapse at once, and gain admission there. Discharged again he would repeat the process at the next hospital, and one day near the end of the war he counted up something like a hundred different post and general hospitals of which he had been an inmate, while he had been admitted to some of them more than half a dozen times each. The surgeons resorted to a variety of expedients by which to get rid of him. They burned his back with hot coppers; gave him the most nauseous mixtures; put him on the lowest possible diet; treated him to cold shower-baths four or five times daily; and did everything else they could think of to drive him from the hospitals, but all to no purpose. In camp it was much the same. On the morning after his arrival from hospital he would wake up with some totally new ache, and report himself upon the sick-list. There was no way by which to conquer his obstinacy, and, as I have said, he escaped duty to the last.

Another curious case, and one which is less easily explained, was that of a much more intelligent man, who for more than a year feigned every conceivable disease, in the hope that he might be discharged the service. One or two of us amused ourselves with his case, by mentioning in his presence the symptoms of some disease of which he had never heard, the surgeon furnishing us the necessary information, and in every case he had the disease within less than twenty-four hours. Finally, and this was the oddest part of the matter, he gave up the attempt, recovered his health suddenly, and became one of the very best soldiers in the battery, a man always ready for duty, and always faithful in its discharge. He was made a corporal and afterwards a sergeant, and there was no better in the battery.

Roberts Bartholomew on Nostalgia

Roberts Bartholomew was a professor at the Medical College of Ohio and served as Assistant Surgeon in the army. The following extract is taken from Bartholomew's 'The Various Influences Affecting the Physical Endurance, the Power of Resisting Disease, etc., of the Men Composing the Volunteer Armies of the United States,' published as Chapter 1 of Austin Flint, ed., *Contributions Relating to the Causes and Prevention of Disease* (1867).

See also: J. Theodore Calhoun, 'Nostalgia as a Disease of Field Service', *Medical and Surgical Reporter* 11 (1864), pp. 130–32; and D.L. and G.T. Anderson, 'Nostalgia and Malingering in the Military during the Civil War', *Perspectives in Biology and Medicine* 28.i (Autumn 1984), pp. 156–66. The term 'nostalgia' was a seventeenth-century coinage applied to soldiers serving in action away from home.

The term nostalgia is derived from two Greek words, signifying, in our vernacular, home-sickness. The derivation of the word indicates the pathology. It is a mental disorder, and belongs to the class melancholia. Certain physical symptoms precede, accompany, or follow the development of the mental aberration: heat of head; increased rapidity of the circulation; constipation; gastro-intestinal disorders of various kinds; a low febrile state simulating typhoid. The mental despondency and the exaltation of the imaginative faculty increase with the decline in the physical strength. Weeping, sighing, groaning, and a constant yearning for home; hallucinations and sometimes maniacal delirium, are the particular forms in which the disorder of the brain expresses itself.

Does the mental state precede the development of the physical symptoms? Is this sufficient of itself to produce that train of gastro-intestinal disorders and febrile phenomena which characterize the progress of the case? My own experience leads me to the conclusion that derangement of the health, particularly of the primary assimilation, leads to the disorders of intellect, and that in those cases in which the affection of the mind precedes the physical disorders, there is much reason to suspect a predisposition to mental derangement to have existed. These questions are not without interest in view of the causes and degree of prevalence of nostalgia during the war. The primal cause is, undoubtedly, absence from home in new and strange surroundings. Various authors have affected to discover a cause in the character of the new country. Thus it is said that the inhabitants of mountainous districts are more prone to home-sickness than the denizen of the plain. The experience of the war hardly confirms this view of the influence of external nature. Both in the first and second year of the war, the number of reported cases were in a precise ratio to the number of troops employed. There was no difference, as far as the statistics show, between the troops on the Atlantic coast and those in the interior region as to the prevalence of nostalgia. Hence it may be assumed that the face of the country in which the troops operated had no influence in the production of this disease.

The cases which occurred under my observation were derived from two classes: young men of feeble will, highly developed imaginative faculties, and strong sexual desires; married men, for the first time absent from their families. The monotony of winter camps favored the development of the peculiar mental and physical effects of nostalgia, whilst active campaigning prevented their occurrence. Having too often no physical nor mental occupation, the minds of these unfortunates reverted homeward. They fell into reverie, and allowed their imaginations to run riot amid the images of home conjured up. Then followed melancholia, hallucinations, and physical phenomena due to disorder of the nervous system, such as borborygmi, constipation, indigestion, irregular action of the heart, disturbed sleep, etc. This interdependence of the morbid physical state upon the mental was rather exceptional. Some derangement of the health in the main, preceded the mental phenomena. According to my observation, deranged sexual functions were more frequently precedent to the mental changes than any other single physical condition. Masturbation and spermatorrhoea produced a mental state more favorable to nostalgia than any other cause. This relation may not be expressed numerically, but if the history of the 2588 cases could be arrived at, the intimacy of the relation existing would be surprising.

Medical Welfare Begins

The following is 'Debut and Prospectus,' from the first issue of *The Crutch* ('A Weekly News and Literary Paper Devoted to the Interest of the Soldier'), which was published weekly by the Annapolis General Hospital, January 1864 to May 1865. From Maryland State Archives. *The Knapsack* was a paper edited by a corps of nurses directed by the surgeon B.A. Vanderkieft, who gave the editors of *The Crutch* a free hand in selecting and reprinting articles of interest. In addition to articles, the paper published news announcements, hospital visiting hours, advertisements for medical products, and correspondence.

In making our first appearance among the great throng of the public journals of the day, it is incumbent upon us to say why we appear, and so give some idea of what we have in view in so appearing – in other words, it is expected of us to display our prospectus, and give the course we purpose pursuing, and then we may have the privilege of asking of a discerning and generous public, a support equal to what it may deem commensurate with the merit of our effort.

In the first place therefore, it is our intention to make the *Crutch* a general directory of all the Hospitals of the Medical Department of Annapolis; to give a general outline of the offices, and officers connected with the post; the commander, officers in charge of the different Hospitals, and the different boards that may be in session at the time of publications, or in prospect of convention.

We purpose it shall contain a complete register of all officers and men, admitted to the Hospital for treatment; of all who return to duty; of all who are discharged from services; of all who leave on furloughs; of all deaths. It will contain also, all circulars, and orders, in relation to furloughs, and leaves of absence; and other circulars, and orders, of general interest, either emanating from this Hospital or this department. In a word, it is our intention to make it a complete HOSPITAL GUIDE for residents or strangers visiting the Hospital, as well as for persons who have friends in, or business with the Hospitals of this district, to enable them to see at a glance, what course will be necessary, in furtherance, either of the object of their visit or communication.

In the second place we desire to make it as far as practicable, a literary and current NEWS JOURNAL. In addition to editorials, it will contain original contributions, and communications, and selections from the best authors, as well as copious extracts from the *Knapsack*, a literary, and humorous paper, edited by the Ladies in connection with the VANDERKIEFT Literary Association of this Hospital, and from other public journals, and a summary of the best news, and the operations of the army.

Thirdly, we desire to make it also beneficial to the soldier personally, by relieving the tedium of a Hospital life, by giving variety to its monotony; by strengthening his interest for good reading, and producing subjects for thought and consideration; and by eliciting, and encouraging his intellectual powers, by offering an opportunity to display them. And lastly, but not the least worthy of notice – we desire to make it a source of pleasure and satisfaction to his friends at home, by giving them constant evidence of his safety, and, at least, the temporal providence that surround him.

It will be seen then that we have a very extensive field before us, and object in view – an object of information, interest and guidance to the public at large – an object of benefiting the soldiers in the Hospital; and an object of pleasure and satisfaction to his friends at home.

To sum up – we hope to make it a readable paper – fit for the fireside or the field – comprensive [*sic*] as well to the young as to the old – and eminently worthy of the confidence, encouragement, and support that we now ask for it.

A comparable publication was *The Cripple*, published 1864–65 by the US General Hospital HQ at Alexandria, Virginia. The issue for November 19, 1864 published the following poem by 'Sanatosia'.

Wounded

Am I awake! Or is it but a dream?
Why, am I here upon the hard damp ground?
Why do I so weak and nerveless seem?
Why is all so dark and still around?

Where are my comrades? – have they left me here?
Can they have fled in fear the battle's tide?
No! they must yet be somewhere by me near.
I'll rise – ha! why this sharp pain in my side!

Ah! I remember now – the rebel traitors came,
And with stout heart we fought them long and well.
But in the midst of battle, smoke and flame
A whizzing bullet struck me and I fell.

But who lies here beside me, prone and still?
With hands and garments stained in gory red,
His life-blood for his country he has spilled.
His eyes are closed – he breathes not, he is dead.

But, ah! I feel my griping wound again.
It's gnawing at my vitals, and my breath
Comes thick and heavy, with the torturing pain.
Oh! Can it be that this will end in death?

And, do I fear to die? No! Life is sweet;
But yet how glorious *thus* one's life to yield.
Still, oh, how dreary, *here* alone to meet
The grim death-angel on the battle-field.

Would you were with me, mother, sisters, now,
That I might see your *dear, loved* forms again.
That your soft hands might cool my fevered brow;
And your kind voices soothe away my pain.

Dear mother, little think you that tonight
Your boy lies helpless, praying you to come,
Else would you, with a fond affection's might,
To cheer his longing heart, leave friends and home.

I'm very weak! This pain o'ertasks my strength.
I'm fainting! oh – we fought them long and well,
And *victory* shall be ours at length – at length –
I'm going! – mother – comrades – all, farewell!

*****

Thus, as he swooned, they found him
At the early dawn of day,
When Life's fast ebbing fountain
Had almost passed away.

(National Library of Medicine transcription)

(Dis)embodied Identities:
Civil War Soldiers, Surgeons,
and the Medical Memories of Combat

Susan-Mary Grant (Newcastle University)

Writing to her mother from Virginia in the summer of 1862, Civil War nurse Katharine Prescott Wormeley described the men under her care as presenting 'a piteous sight.' No one, she went on, 'knows what war is until they see this black side of it.' She reassured her mother, however, that it was not all misery. 'We see the dark side of all. You must not, however, gather only gloomy ideas from me. I see the worst,' she wrote, 'short of the actual battle-field, that there is to see.'[1]

What Wormeley did see was grim. She described 'four or five amputations. One poor fellow,' she reported, had been 'shot through the knee,' and was 'enduring more than mortal agony; a fair-haired boy of seventeen,' had been 'shot through the lungs, every breath he draws hissing through the wound.' She noted, too, that it was not the wounds that posed the greatest threat to life on the James Peninsula in the spring of 1862, but 'the terrible decimating diseases brought on by exposure and hardships and the climate of marshes and watercourses.' And the physical effects were hardly the worst of it. Anyone, she observed, who 'sees the suffering, despondent attitudes of the men, and their worn frames and faces, knows what war is, better than the sight of wounds can teach it.' Wormeley was especially distressed by several cases of attempted suicide that she encountered; soldiers so destroyed by their experiences that they were 'out of their minds.' One had tried to drown himself three times. Yet, for Wormeley, the maimed bodies and the suffering she witnessed and struggled to alleviate neither dampened her dedication to

1 Katharine Prescott Wormeley to mother, May 26 and June 10, 1862, in Katharine Prescott Wormeley, *The Other Side of War* (Boston: Ticknor and Company, 1889, second edition; orig. 1888), pp. 77, 131.

her work nor undermined her support for the Union cause. '*This is life,*' she enthused in the midst of death.[2]

The Cruel Side of War

The eventual publication of Wormeley's letters from the James Peninsula in 1888 was designed, as its title made clear, to highlight *The Other Side of War*. But there was an ambiguity in this title. 'Other' could refer to the medical challenges that the war posed; equally, it could simply have referred to the work of Union nurses, a reminder that women, as well as men, had played their part in the Civil War. A decade later, however, when the United States found itself at war with Spain, any ambiguity was dispelled by the new title accorded the 1898 version of her volume: *The Cruel Side of War*.

Reviewing Wormeley's work, the *New York Times* reassured its readers that the medical problems that Wormeley had encountered were a thing of the past. 'In those days,' it advised its readers, 'carbolic acid was scarcely understood, iodoform did not exist, listerine was yet to be discovered, and a physician would sooner have beheaded a patient than have bandaged a wound and left it untouched for days depending upon nature and bichloride of mercury to heal it. Vaseline, cosmolene, agnino, lanine, all the coal-oil and wool-product ointments were yet to be discovered, and the science of antiseptic surgery was unborn.'[3]

For the *New York Times*, the cruel side of the Civil War inhered in medical ignorance, both sanitary and surgical. Following this reasoning, it was simply the Civil War soldier's misfortune that the war was located before – tragically just before – the start of the narrative of modern medical progress and performance inaugurated by Joseph Lister's publication 'On the Antiseptic Principle in the Practice of Surgery' (1867). Lister's use of carbolic acid, as the *New York Times* noted, and his discovery of its efficacy in dealing with compound fractures 'in which the effects of decomposition in the injured part were especially striking and pernicious' came just too late to benefit Civil War troops. As a consequence, Civil War medical care is regarded not as a chapter in the story of medicine's development but rather as a closed book whose contents hardly bear contemplation.[4]

2   Wormeley to mother, May 13 and May 14, and to 'Friend,' May 16 and May 11, 1862, *Other Side of War*, pp. 25–26, 34–35, 38, 19; emphasis in original.
3   'War and Navies: Miss Wormeley's Volume on the Cruel Side of War,' *New York Times*, April 16, 1898.
4   Joseph Lister, 'On the Antiseptic Principle in the Practice of Surgery,' *British*

But this conceptual chronological continuum can be misleading. As the noted neurologist Silas Weir Mitchell commented, science 'is forever changing. The work of today is contradicted tomorrow.' And Civil War surgeons were obviously unaware at the time that they were operating in 'the very last years of the medical middle ages.' Even as Wormeley wrote her letters from Virginia, the *American Medical Times* anticipated that the conflict's 'influence upon the progress of military, naval, and medical sciences' would be 'deemed worthy of record.' Few, it was believed, would recall 'its bad surgery; the limbs wantonly sacrificed; the lives lost that would have been saved by timely operations; the unseemly incisions; the careless dressings; the neglect of medical treatment.' The cruel side of the Civil War, the paper argued, would simply fade away, and 'quietly seek the oblivion of the grave.'[5]

The fact that the opposite was actually the case, and that it was the war's 'influence upon the progress of military, naval, and medical sciences' that faded from professional and public memory alike owed something to timing, certainly, but also to hindsight. A surgeon such as William Williams Keen, for example, whose career had begun during the Civil War but spanned the First World War a half century later (Keen died in 1932), could not help but compare his early professional experiences against the developments in medical knowledge, in equipment, and especially in the understanding of antisepsis and asepsis, that occurred over his lifetime. His 'Surgical Reminiscences of the Civil War,' a lecture delivered in 1905 to the College of Physicians of Philadelphia, effectively comprised a catalogue of the medical incompetence, ignorance, and incomprehension that pertained between 1861 and 1865. He recalled, for example, the ineptitude of one brigade surgeon who had been asked to 'compress the subclavian artery' in the course of aiding an amputation, but who had instead applied 'vigorous pressure' below, rather than above the clavicle, causing a haemorrhage that Keen was, thankfully, able to control.[6]

Medical Journal 2 (1867), p. 246 at http://www.ncbi.nlm.nih.gov/pmc/articles/PMC2895849/ (February 1, 2015); for a discussion of contemporary reactions to Civil War medicine, see Susan-Mary Grant, '"*Mortal* in this *season*": Union Surgeons and the Narrative of Medical Modernisation in the American Civil War,' *Social History of Medicine* 27.iv (November 2014), pp. 689–707.

5   S. Weir Mitchell, 'Biographical Memoir of John Shaw Billings,' in *Biographical Memoirs* (Washington: National Academy of Sciences, 1917), Vol. III, p. 383; George Worthington Adams, 'Confederate Medicine,' *The Journal of Southern History* 6:ii (May 1940), pp. 151–66, quotation 151; anon, 'A Remedy for an Evil,' *American Medical Times*, June 14, 1862, p. 335.

6   William Williams Keen, 'Surgical Reminiscences of the Civil War,' in *Addresses*

'The surgery of that time,' Keen recounted, 'was very simple – cold water dressings or simple cerate [a wax ointment] spread on lint made by patriotic women by scraping one side of old linen sheets or tablecloths, or, to encourage suppuration (for pus at that time could be "laudable"), the ordinary flaxseed poultice. An amputation stump was always dressed with a Maltese cross of lint spread with cerate,' with ligatures securing the arteries, Keen recalled, and the risk of secondary haemorrhage was high. Worse was the risk of infection. In the absence of antiseptics, hospital gangrene was rife; some 45 percent of those who contracted it died. 'Often did I see a simple gunshot wound, scarcely larger than the bullet which made it,' Keen remembered, 'become larger and larger until a hand would scarce cover it, and extend from the skin downward into the tissues until one could put half his fist into the sloughing wound.'[7]

Keen noted that were such cases to present themselves in 1905, they would most likely be recognised as a 'streptococcus infection,' but in the mid-1860s no such diagnosis was possible. And amputation was not necessarily the cause, although the procedure certainly rendered infection more likely and was more common during the Civil War than it would later become. 'Conservative treatment of joints was,' as Keen observed, 'an impossibility until antisepsis and asepsis made it not only a possibility, but a duty.' And although he argued – as did many of the leading surgeons who served during the war – that 'far more lives were lost from refusal to amputate than by amputation,' the mortality figures from that as from other procedures were sobering.[8]

On Keen's figures alone, out of '852 amputations at the shoulder-joint, 236 died, a mortality of 28.5 per cent. Of 66 cases of amputation of the hip-joint 55, or 83.3 per cent., died. Of 155 cases of trephining, 60 recovered and 95 died, a mortality of over 61 per cent. Of 374 ligations of the femoral artery, 93 recovered and 281 died, a mortality of over 75 per cent [...] These figures,' he observed, 'afford a striking evidence of the dreadful mortality of military surgery in the days before antisepsis and first-aid packages.' Placed within the wider context of the lack of medical and indeed military organisation at the start of the war, shortages of food as well as medical supplies, and absence of suitable hospital and transport facilities for the wounded, it may be no surprise that Keen concluded, from the perspective of 1905, that '[w]hat we did not have in those days was almost more noticeable than what we did have.'[9]

and Other Papers (Philadelphia: W.B. Saunders and Company, 1905), pp. 420–41, 422.

7   Keen, 'Surgical Reminiscences,' pp. 429, 430–31, 432.
8   Keen, 'Surgical Reminiscences,' p. 430.
9   Keen, 'Surgical Reminiscences,' pp. 433–34.

This anachronistic observation has informed the discussion of Civil War medicine well beyond 1905. But hindsight made Keen too harsh on his younger self. In his professional capacity as a Union surgeon, Keen was instrumental in mitigating, albeit inadequately by his own later lights, the wounds of the Civil War. In the process he, and his colleagues, paved the way not just for the professionalization of medicine in the United States, but for a body of publications detailing their surgical successes and failures alike, intended for, and used by, future generations of surgeons. One of the works he published, together with George R. Morehouse and Silas Weir Mitchell – *Gunshot Wounds and other Injuries of Nerves* (1864) – was still in use during the First World War, when Keen himself published, at the age of seventy-nine, *The Treatment of War Wounds* (1917). But perhaps one of the most impressive publications that he contributed to in the course of his career was the multi-volume *Medical and Surgical History of the War of the Rebellion* (*MSHWR*).[10]

A composite work, whose publication was directed by the then Surgeon General of the United States Army, Joseph K. Barnes, the original six volumes of the *MSHWR* were almost two decades in the making. The end result comprised the reports and case-notes of many individual doctors, accompanied by statistical reports and tables and a wealth of images of Civil War soldiers, the wounds they sustained and the treatment they received. The significance accorded the *MSHWR* at the time, however, has not always been acknowledged by subsequent generations.

Although the very existence of the *MSHWR* rather disproved poet Walt Whitman's famous assertion that 'the real war will never get in the books,' the public, and indeed some scholars, have tended to prefer the fictional over the factual as far as Civil War wounds are concerned. Only through the literary voice, it has been argued, can we hear the language of the damaged, physical body.[11] Yet this is where the *MSHWR* is especially valuable. Because although conceived as a mainly medical publication, both 'a contribution to science' and 'an enduring monument to the self-sacrificing zeal and professional ability of the Volunteer and Regular Medical Staff' of the Union army, the *MSHWR* was arguably much more than a patriotic, professional publication.

---

10   Joseph K. Barnes (ed.), *The Medical and Surgical History of the War of the Rebellion between 1870 and 1880* (hereinafter *MSHWR*), 6 vols (Washington, DC: US Government Printing Office, 1870–88).

11   Walt Whitman, *Specimen Days and Collect* (1883, reprint; New York: Dover Publications, 1995), p. 80; David T. Mitchell and Sharon L. Snyder, *Narrative Prosthesis: Disability and the Dependencies of Discourse* (Ann Arbor, MI: University of Michigan Press, 2001), p. 64.

It became, in fact, a multi-layered, textured, textual voice for and of the Civil War wounded.[12]

Few of those wounded could record their trauma in their own words, of course. A notable exception was Lieutenant J. Edmund Mallet of the 81st New York Infantry, who provided posterity with a dramatic account not just of the immediate physical sensations he experienced when shot but of his long road to recovery. 'I distinctly remember the sensations experienced upon being hit,' Mallet recorded:

> I imagined that a cannon ball had struck me on the left hip-bone, that it took a downward course, tearing the intestines in its course, and lodged against the marrow of the right thigh-bone. I fancied I saw sparks of fire, and curtains of cobwebs wet with dew, sparkling in the sun. I heard a monotonous roar as of distant cataracts. I felt my teeth chatter, a rush of blood to my eyes, ears, nose, and to the ends of my fingers and toes. These sensations crowded themselves in the instants in which I struggled to stand, and actually fell forward on my face. As I fell, I experienced another sensation as of a sudden and violent blow on the nape of the neck, and then became completely insensible.[13]

Mallet was unusually articulate about the entire process of being wounded. The experience of most soldiers as that appears in the *MSHWR* can be accessed only second-hand, in the case-notes provided by their surgeons. Nevertheless, through these we can discern not just the language of physical destruction but that of reconstruction; not just confirmation of the cruel side of war, but evidence of the contemporary medical battle against war's cruelty; and proof not just of the soldiers' suffering, but of the struggle for their survival.

The (Re)Constructive Side of War

For the fledgling American medical profession the 'clinics of the battlefield' represented an opportunity to be seized. Those who, like Keen, were at the start of their careers in 1861 saw the Civil War as a means of acquiring the crucial practical skills required to bolster their theoretical training. John Shaw Billings, who became one of the war's foremost surgeons but had only graduated in 1860, brought to the front some of the latest medical equipment, including a 'set of clinical thermometers [...] a hypodermic syringe, and a

12 Joseph K. Barnes, introduction to *MSHWR*, Part I, Vol. 1 (1870), p. ix.
13 *MSHWR*, Part II, Vol. II (1876), pp. 90–91.

Symes staff for urethral stricturotomy,' confident that these would help him 'to acquire a reputation and surgical glory.'[14]

Building a reputation was not the only opportunity the war offered. Professional and patriotic pride also came into play. The Medical Director of the Army of the Potomac, Jonathan Letterman, realized that the war provided physicians with a unique opportunity to acquire knowledge that would 'go far toward filling the hiatus which exists in that branch of science in which we are now engaged, that of military surgery.' And for the Medical Director of the Army of the Ohio, Henry S. Hewitt, the sectional schism would produce a national triumph by enabling the United States 'to present the world with the most perfect system of military surgery that has appeared, and make our observation and experience the point of departure and the standard of comparison for the future.'[15]

What was needed, as men such as Letterman, Hewitt, and the newly appointed Surgeon General, William Alexander Hammond, realised, was an authoritative professional record of battlefield surgery. Consequently, under the direction of Hammond, Union surgeons were charged not just with the recording of symptoms and the study of sanitary arrangements during the war, but the acquisition of 'all specimens of morbid anatomy, surgical or medical [...] together with projectiles and foreign bodies removed, and such other matters as may prove of interest in the study of military medicine or surgery' with a view not just to the compiling of what became, in time, the *MSHWR* but the establishment, during the war itself, of the Army Medical Museum

14   Mitchell, 'Memoir of Billings,' p. 376; Fielding H. Garrison, *John Shaw Billings: A Memoir* (New York and London: G.P. Putnam's Sons, 1915), pp. 20–22, 27; see also Billings, 'Medical Reminiscences of the Civil War,' *Transactions of the College of Physicians of Philadelphia*, Vol. 27 (1905), pp.115–21.

15   Jonathan Letterman, memorandum to Corps Medical Directors, April 27, 1863, in Letterman, *Medical Recollections of the Army of the Potomac* (New York: D. Appleton and Company, 1866), pp. 114–15; 'Report of Surg. Henry S. Hewitt, US Army, Medical Director, Department of the Ohio, May, 1 – September 8, 1864 (Atlanta Campaign), January 1865,' *Official Records of the War of the Rebellion* (OR) Series I, Vol. XXXVIII/2, p. 534. A great many medical reports apart from the *MSHWR* came out of the war; see, for example, Frank Hasting Hamilton (ed.), Stephen Smith, M.D., *Analysis of Four Hundred and Thirty-Nine Recorded Amputations in the Contiguity of the Lower Extremity*; and Joseph Jones, MD, *Investigations Upon the Nature, Causes, and Treatment of Hospital Gangrene, as it Prevailed in the Confederate Armies, 1861–1865* (Cambridge, MA: Kurd and Houghton, Riverside Press for the United States Sanitary Commission, 1871).

(AMM). 'It is scarcely necessary,' Hammond argued in the summer of 1862, 'to remind the medical officers of the regular and volunteer services that through the means in question much may be done to advance the science which we all have so much at heart,' and he 'confidently expected' that no Civil War surgeon would 'neglect this opportunity of advancing the honor of the service, the cause of humanity, and his own reputation.'[16]

A surgeon such as Keen needed no prompting in this regard. Appointed by John H. Brinton, who had been put in charge of the AMM, Keen recalled that it had been his 'duty to gather and forward [to the AMM] all the specimens that I could lay hands upon.' Reactions to this initiative were mixed, however. Union general Daniel E. Sickles famously dispatched his leg, amputated after the Battle of Gettysburg, to the new museum, and was said to have visited it on an annual basis after the war. Indeed, as the famous author Mark Twain observed many years later, Sickles 'valued his lost leg above the one that is left. I am perfectly sure,' Twain mused, 'that if he had to part with either of them he would part with the one that he has got.' Others were less enthusiastic, however, at the idea that, having lost a part of themselves to the Union war effort, that part might end up in the AMM. Brinton himself recalled the vigorous opposition he had met with from a soldier whose amputated limb Brinton had selected as a suitable museum specimen. Challenged, 'noisily and pertinaciously,' to return the limb to its former owner, Brinton refused on the grounds that since the soldier had signed up for three years he still had time left to serve. Consequently, Brinton declared, the government was 'entitled to all of [him], until the expiration of the specified time. I dare not give a part of you up before,' Brinton told him. 'Come, *then*, and you can have the rest of you, but not before.'[17]

16   William A. Hammond, *Circular No. 2, May 21, 1862* (Washington, DC: Surgeon General's Office, 1862). On the origins and development of the Army Medical Museum see Robert S. Henry, *The Armed Forces Institute of Pathology, Its First Century, 1862–1962* (Washington, DC: Office of the Surgeon General, Department of the Army, 1964), esp. Chapters 1–3. The remit for the medical museum collections was expanded in 1863 to include requests for photographic representations of wounds; see Stanley B. Burns, M.D., *Shooting Soldiers: Civil War Medical Photography by R.B. Bontecou* (New York: The Burns Archive, 2011), p. 16; Hammond, *Circular No. 5, June 9, 1862* (Washington, DC: Surgeon General's Office, 1862).

17   Keen, 'Surgical Reminiscences,' p. 433; Mark Twain, *Autobiography of Mark Twain*, edited Harriet Elinor Smith (Berkeley, CA: University of California Press, 2010), p. 289; John H. Brinton, *Personal Memoirs of John H. Brinton, Civil*

Rank and file military opposition to some medical initiatives notwith-standing, it soon became 'quite evident,' as one correspondent to the medical journal *Cincinnati Lancet and Observer* noted, 'that since this unholy warfare commenced, military surgery has received such an impetus in this country that hereafter it will form an important part in the medical literature of the age.' The Civil War, it was noted, had opened 'a wide field of observation, from which surgery gathers its rich and varied laurels. The destructive missiles of war are becoming our teachers,' it was observed, 'for in proportion as they mutilate the more important tissues of the body, so is the skill of our art taxed to repair the injury inflicted.' And by the war's end, one serving surgeon highlighted the great 'improvement [that] has been made in the art of surgery during the last few years, particularly since this war has taken place.'[18]

These were not unrealistic claims at the time. The wealth of cases documented in the *MSHWR* reveal the extent and complexity – and indeed the success rates – of many of the surgical operations undertaken during the war. But the popular understanding of Civil War surgery has, in the century and a half since the war, been too readily reduced to one specific procedure: amputation. That this was an important aspect of Civil War medical treatment is without doubt. One notable case was that of Columbus Rush, a Confederate soldier from Georgia, who lost both legs and was fitted with prosthetic limbs by Erasmus Darwin Hudson, the leading Union surgeon in extremity prosthetics, which enabled him to walk again (see Plates 3 and 4). Another was that of Union soldier Charles N. Lapham, also successfully fitted with artificial limbs by Hudson (see Plates 5 and 6). Just over a year after his legs had been shattered by solid shot and amputated, Lapham was able to walk again and even climb stairs.[19]

Mobility and individual recovery were, of course, not the only issues as far as war wounds were concerned. The political, social, and economic mileage that men such as Columbus Rush and Dan Sickles derived from their missing

---

War Surgeon, 1861–1865 (1891, reprint; Carbondale and Edwardsville: Southern Illinois University Press, 1996), p. 54.

18   *Cincinnati Lancet and Observer*, February 1863, pp. 107–9; Wm. B. McGarvan, Surgeon, Twenty-Sixth Ohio Volunteer Infantry, 'Amputation of Left Arm at the Shoulder Joint, and Resection of the Head of the Right Humerus,' *Cincinnati Lancet and Observer*, May 1865, pp. 276–78.

19   See Columbus Rush to Hudson in Blair O. Rogers, 'Rehabilitation of Wounded Civil War Veterans,' *Aesthetic Plastic Surgery*, 26 (2002): 498-519, 507; *MSHRW*, Part III, Vol. 2, 224-225; Figs. 176 and 177 from AMM photographs 154, 155.

limbs – which served both as potent reminders of the part they had played in the war, and valuable physical evidence for future pension claims – should not, of course, be underestimated. Because as Mark Twain noted, Sickles was not alone in his attachment to a missing limb. Twain cited the example of General Lucius Fairchild from Wisconsin, who had lost an arm, also at Gettysburg. '[W]henever a proper occasion' presented itself, he observed, one that gave him 'an opportunity to elevate the stump of the lost arm and wag it with effect [...] that is what he did.'

Although Fairchild clearly eschewed an artificial limb, many, like Rush, did not. The dramatic growth of the prosthetic limb industry in the years following the war informed more than medical science; it spoke to the emergent man/machine imperatives of a modernising nation in which everything and everyone could be streamlined, rendered new, and improved by science. So as a rehabilitative, reconstructive trope, applicable alike to the individual and the nation, the science of prosthesis has extensive intellectual interrogative mileage, certainly. But both contemporary and subsequent fascination with this aspect of Civil War medicine disguises more than it reveals about its surgical side.

One of the least-appreciated aspects of Civil War reconstructive surgery, although carefully detailed in the *MSHWR*, was its plastic surgery successes. Although plastic surgery techniques were practiced by only a handful of surgeons during the Civil War, including Keen, the importance of the procedure to those who had suffered facial injuries, especially, cannot be underestimated. One of the few, but arguably the most skilful as far as reparative autoplastic techniques at the time was concerned, was New York surgeon Gurdon Buck, one of the founders of the New York Academy of Medicine and author of the first American study of plastic surgery, *Contributions to Reparative Surgery* (1876). He was also one of the pioneers in the use of medical photography to facilitate surgeons' understanding and treatment of war wounds.

In the year after the Civil War ended, Buck published one of his cases, that of a young soldier – he was just twenty years old – William Simmons, from the New York Heavy Infantry regiment. Struck by a shell outside Petersburg toward the end of the war, Simmons lost most of his lower jaw, rendering him incapable of mastication and making speech extremely difficult. Buck was forced to reconstruct by simply restructuring Simmons' face, but did so in such a way as to effect '[s]ome improvement in the general appearance and expression of his face, as well as in articulation.' Simmons was 'able to maintain his lips in contact and thus prevent the escape of the saliva,' which were, Buck noted, 'the important results achieved by this successful operation, equally gratifying to the patient and satisfying to the surgeon.' Before long,

Simmons had his voice back, and 'no longer showed any reluctance to engage in conversation.'[20]

One of Buck's most complicated cases, however, and one that involved five separate operations over several months and a skin-graft, had nothing to do with the devastating effects of Civil War weaponry, but was rather the result of medication; or more accurately over-medication, seemingly mercury prescribed for typhoid fever, that had resulted in a devastating and destructive form of osteonecrosis of the jaw. Carleton Burgan was, like Simmons, only twenty years old when, thanks to Keen – who wrote up the preliminary notes for the case – he came to Buck's attention, having been discharged from the army on medical grounds. With the aid of Thomas B. Gunning, a dentist, Burgan underwent extensive and lengthy (one operation took three hours) surgery to reconstruct his damaged face (see Plates 7 and 8; see also Plates 9 and 10 for a similar operation done on a Private Rowland Ward). Prosthetic nose and removable upper-jaw pieces were constructed by Gunning from vulcanite, both being necessary, as Buck explained, to 'supply the place of the lost maxillary bone, and afford a solid support that would have to be transposed for the reconstruction of the mouth and the closure of the cheeks and nostrils,' but also to enable Burgan to breathe properly. Crucial to the success of the operations – and a reminder that not all Civil War surgeons were unaware of the complications of contagion – was that Burgan was 'placed in an outbuilding on the hospital premises which had not been in use for several weeks, and where he and his attendants would be the sole occupants.'[21]

Ultimately, as Buck acknowledged, it was impossible fully to repair the dreadful damage that Burgan's face had sustained, but, as in Simmons' case, he was able to give Burgan his life, and his voice back. Prior to the surgery, Buck noted, Burgan had been 'scarcely intelligible.' Visiting his former patient several years later, he was gratified to discover that he was well, had married and had two children (Burgan would go on to have eight), and was working. In later life, Burgan took to wearing a leather flap over the damaged side of his face, suggesting that he remained self-conscious about the face he brought home from the Civil War, the one he now had to face life with. But it was a relatively

20   Gurdon Buck, *Case of Destruction of the Body of the Lower Jaw and Extensive Disfiguration of the Face from a Shell Wound* (Albany: Private Printing, 1866), pp. 4–5.
21   William W. Keen, 'Gangrene of the Face Following Salivation,' National Museum of Army Medicine Accession File 1000867; Gurdon Buck, *Contributions to Reparative Surgery* (New York: D. Appleton and Company, 1876), pp. 36, 38.

long life – Burgan was seventy-two when he died – and one he might not have had without the skill of Gurdon Buck.[22]

Conclusion

The evidence of several successful cases does not, of course, contradict the fact that Civil War medical treatment was, in many respects, an appalling and frequently terminal experience for all concerned. But the medical memories of the Civil War have been skewed by subsequent medical developments. A surgeon such as Keen, whose long career provided its own comparative perspective, perhaps dwelt too much on the 'dreadful things' that Civil War surgeons 'did do' and the 'good things' that they 'did not dare to do.'[23] But this retrospective regret, although fully understandable, has sometimes led to the wrong questions being asked of Civil War medical procedures and practices, and to a reluctance to engage fully with the evidence provided by medical sources such as the *MSHWR*.

Yet there may be another reason why we veer away from the Civil War's medical memories, one that draws together rather than divides the nineteenth century from the twenty-first. Because although Keen argued, in 1905, that the terrible mortality figures from the Civil War 'can never again be seen, at least in civilized warfare,' he was ultimately equivocal about medicine's ability to civilise war beyond a certain point. No 'matter what progress is made in the scientific treatment of wounds' he noted, warfare was suffering.[24]

Keen's sobering suggestion that modern, mass warfare was never going to be able to provide the level of support required by soldiers in the field reminds us that we should beware of being too complacent about the scientific strides taken in the century and a half between the Civil War and our own time. Too often we look to the Civil War for reassurance that the present represents an improvement over the past as far as the treatment of and reaction to wounded soldiers is concerned. We seek social as well as historical inclusion for the wounded, and for the warrior, whose voices are often deemed to have been 'forgotten' by societies, past and present, careless of their sacrifice. But in the process of normalising the wounds of war in the world beyond the battlefield, we still struggle to include both soldier and surgeon within that world. Too often, we abandon the wounded veteran to a medical discourse that remains socially and scientifically distinct. The bodies of the Civil War wounded as

22   Buck, *Contributions to Reparative Surgery*, p. 50.
23   Keen, 'Surgical Reminiscences,' pp. 433–34.
24   Keen, 'Surgical Reminiscences,' p. 441.

detailed in the many and varied memories – personal and professional, literary and medical, visual and visceral – of that conflict speak to the need for a more inclusive narrative, one that brings together the medical and the martial, the soldier and the surgeon; one that fully embodies the essence of modern war.

PHOTOGRAPHY

Painful Looks:
Reading Civil War Photographs

Mick Gidley (University of Leeds)

As soon as the Civil War broke out, photographers were on the scene. Mathew B. Brady, the leading photographic entrepreneur of the time – someone who in his project to produce and sell a *Gallery of Illustrious Americans* (1850) had already demonstrated the medium's capacity to intersect with history – set off, with assistants, alongside part of the advancing Union army. One of the stories that soon attached itself to his name – he assiduously promoted such tales – is that in the confusion of the early indecisive battle now known as Bull Run (1861) he was lost in the woods for three whole days. On Brady's return to New York, the newspapers claimed that he had salvaged from his wanderings a trove of exact transcriptions of the battlefield – but, if he did, none survived. In any case, his eyesight had so deteriorated by this point that it is unlikely he took such pictures himself. He also sent operatives into the field equipped with dark-room wagons, their cameras, chemicals, and plates aboard, ready to make wet-plate images, and much of these photographers' output was copyrighted and circulated under Brady's name. Throughout the war, and for a while afterwards, he mounted exhibitions of such photographs in his Manhattan gallery.[1]

It is important to realize that, primarily for technical reasons, the battlefield photographs were not made during the heat of combat. They were taken days, weeks, sometimes months after the fighting at that location had ceased.[2] The resulting images are not so much records of events as reflections

---

1   For more on Brady, see Mary Panzer, *Mathew Brady and the Image of History* (Washington, DC, and London: Smithsonian Institution Press for the National Portrait Gallery, 1997).

2   William A. Frassanito, notably in *Gettysburg: A Journey in Time* (New York:

upon events. Sometimes the composition itself tells us this. The well-known view (initially attributed to Brady but actually taken by one of his assistants) often titled 'McPerson's Woods – Wheatfields in which General Reynolds was Shot' shows Brady himself surveying the Gettysburg battlefield scene in 1863. He acts as a surrogate viewer: we look at him – tellingly across a reflecting pool – as he contemplates the spot where a sniper's bullet took down the Union commander John Reynolds (see Plate 11). We fill the prospect with our thoughts. Uncaptioned, this image would constitute a rural scene, but its title animates it differently. To their original viewers, such landscapes were haunted by the deadly events that had occurred there. All of the photographs we are considering here were an aftermath of the war.

* * *

Within weeks of the war's onset, the Army of the Potomac, on the Union side, had issued as many as 300 permits to itinerant photographers. Such men would camp close to the lines, advertise their facilities, and then make inexpensive tintype likenesses for individual soldiers to send to their families, friends, and sweethearts back home. All too many such portraits ultimately became mementos of their fallen subjects. That the presence of these opportunist cameramen became well known lends credibility to E.L. Doctorow's decision, in his novel *The March* (2005), to disguise a would-be Southern assassin as an itinerant photographer and to let him follow General William Tecumseh Sherman's army as it laid waste to the South during the famous march, in the autumn of 1864, from Atlanta to the sea.[3]

While for some photographers the war constituted an unexpected opportunity, others were thoroughly prepared for it. The military hierarchy generally appreciated the medium and, even ahead of the war, specific units of the army made extensive use of it. The Topographical Engineering Corps, for

Scribner's Sons, 1975) and *Antietam: The Photographic Legacy of America's Bloodiest Day* (New York: Charles Scribner's Sons, 1978), has carefully established firm timelines for the photographs. By contrast, artists at the battle front, such as the young Winslow Homer, were able to draw scenes of action almost as they happened, and the results appeared as engravings in the illustrated press.

3   One of the best compendiums of Civil War photographs – including tintype portraits – is the book that accompanied Ken and Ric Burns' ten-hour film documentary, *The Civil War*: Geoffrey C. Ward, *The Civil War: An Illustrated History* (London: The Bodley Head, 1991); E.L. Doctorow, *The March* (orig. 2005; London: Abacus, 2006).

example, formally employed photographers to make maps, battlefield diagrams, and the like. Andrew J. Russell – who in the decade after the war would make hundreds of photographs for the Union Pacific Railroad as it laid ever more miles of track into the West – developed his skills largely through working closely with General Herman Haupt, the innovative head of the US Bureau of Military Railroads. He made images that would become illustrations in Haupt's practical guide for staff officers, *Military Bridges*, published in 1863. In the same year, with a more general remit as an official army photographer, Russell photographed armaments and assembled troops ahead of the battles at Chancellorsville and Fredricksburg.[4]At Fredricksburg, in a brief interlude in the fighting, before the ground on which he stood was re-taken by the Confederates, he took a photograph of dead Confederate artilliery horses and battered ammunition carriers (see Plate 12). In this image, the concern with looking that I see as characteristic of so many Civil War photographs is made explicit: General Haupt leans against a shattered tree stump, surveying the destruction below him, two other figures gaze around them, and we, too, look at the felled animals and the upturned vehicles.

George N. Barnard and Alexander Gardner, both former Brady employees, served in a variety of posts during the war. Barnard was official photographer of the Chief Engineer's Office, Division of Mississippi, and accompanied Sherman on the march from Atlanta. Alan Trachtenberg has read the 'narrative' of Barnard's pictures, collected and arranged in *Photographic Views of Sherman's Campaign* (1866), as charting the most naked 'logic of war: destroy the enemy,' and thus sees the book's final images, 'Ruins in Charleston, SC' (see Plate 13) and 'Ruins of the Railroad Depot, Charleston, SC,' not just as records of the North's military victory but as symbolic reflections on the moral failure and fall of the slave South.[5] 'Ruins in Charleston' helpfully includes two contemplative surveyors of the scene, and for the symbolism to work effectively, each image needs careful perusal as the viewer turns the book's pages.

4   A thorough yet succinct account of photography during the Civil War is Keith F. Davis, "'A Terrible Distinctness": Photography of the Civil War Era", in Martha A. Sandweiss, ed., *Photography in Nineteenth-Century America* (New York: Harry N. Abrams for Amon Carter Museum, 1991), pp. 128–79.
5   Alan Trachtenberg, the 'Albums of War' chapter in *Reading American Photographs: Images as History, Mathew Brady to Walker Evans* (New York: Hill and Wang, 1989), pp. 71–118 (quotation p. 99). Barnard's book is available as an inexpensive reprint: George N. Barnard, *Photographic Views of Sherman's Campaign* (New York: Dover, 1977).

Gardner – who in professional skill and business acumen later came to rival Brady – in 1862 was appointed the official photographer for General George McClellan's Army of the Potomac, and, as an honorary captain, served at Warrenton, Antietam, and other battles, making some impressive images. When Lincoln demoted McClellan, Gardner set up his own studio, poached some of Brady's best operatives, and, after acquiring from Brady the rights to both Gardner-made pictures and those of some of his colleagues, sent his own team into the field. At the end of the war, he gathered a selection of such work into the two-volume *Gardner's Photographic Sketch Book of the War* (1866). The *Sketch Book* – which was sold on a subscription basis in an expensive limited edition – constructed, through its combination of collodian prints and extended captions, both a chronological series of stories about the war and an over-arching narrative of the inevitable triumph of the righteous North.[6] We will need to look at at some of its images.

At the onset of the war, the Medical Department of the army was already relying on photography for purposes of documentation and training. The visual symptoms of particular ailments and the effects of injury were almost routinely recorded. Since the war itself produced thousands of casualties and led to a huge rise in communicable diseases – a much greater threat to the life and limb of ill-nourished troops than the enemy's weapons – it gave much work to photographers. Their efforts were thoroughly institutionalised by the establishment, as early as 1862, of the Army Medical Museum, which determined to collect 'all specimens of morbid anatomy, surgical or medical, which may be regarded as valuable; together with projectiles and foreign bodies removed, and such other matters as may prove of interest in the study of military medicine.'[7]

The Museum gathered photographs from way stations, makeshift infirmaries, and newly built hospitals; these depicted nurses and other personnel, gleaming new interiors, operations in progress, portraits of uniformed men with their new crutches, and a large number of close-up views of wounded soldiers (see Plate 14). In these the focus is on the wounds or prosthetic limbs rather than on the men, who often hold blackboards scrawled with their names and service numbers. Titled by wound – 'Shot forearm,' 'Double amputation,' and the like – they show skin sewn like gathered cloth over the sunken space where ribs had been; holes, some see-through, in thighs and upper arms; deep

---

6   The *Sketch Book* is available as an inexpensive reprint: Alexander Gardner, *Gardner's Sketch Book of the Civil War* (New York: Dover, 1959). Trachtenberg has advanced a detailed interpretation of it, making subtle comparison with Barnard's book, in *Reading American Photographs*, pp. 93–111.

7   Official order by the Surgeon General, quoted in Davis, p. 160.

gashes; hanging folds of skin; throats open as mouths; and men legless, armless, or missing half a jaw. What makes them more disturbing is that the men, with their blackboards, seem aquiesent in this objectifying process, even when there are two of them together in the same photograph, as if they are not just giving up their identities, like criminals in mugshots, but abjectly examining themselves in their new state.

The Medical Museum also set up its own photographic department headed by Liverpool-born William H. Bell, a very experienced and accomplished practioner of the medium. He, too, had worked for Brady and after the war, like almost all of the other photographers mentioned by name here, he would head West to make sponsored landscapes. His subject while at the Museum was the landscape of the body. Bell's principal task, as reported by the *Philadelphia Photographer* in 1866, was 'to photograph shattered bones, broken skulls, and living subjects before and after surgical operations have been performed on them.' 'We were shown some photographs of the wounded, before and after surgery had been performed,' the reporter went on, commenting, 'certainly photography is the only medium by which surgery could so plainly make known its handiwork.'[8]

There is, indeed, a purely indexical aspect to Bell's work that proves almost overwhelming. In his 'Gunshot Wound of Left Femur' (1865–67), a straight-on full-length portrait, the concentration, as the picture's title indicates, is on the man's left leg, viewed both directly and as reflected in a mirror the man holds behind him. Whereas in most portraits we look at the sitter's face, especially the eyes, noting anything that seems the least bit unusual, and register the subject's expression, deportment, and dress, here the wound on the man's naked thigh takes our gaze, and the man himself, his shirt roughly folded to conceal his genitals, becomes only its vulnerable bearer. This emphatically does *not* constitute a studio portrait: behind the man there is no pictorial backdrop, just a bare wall. Bell's 'Gunshot Fracture of the Shaft of the Right Femur, United with Great Shortening and Deformity' (1865) is also not a studio portrait, but in a different way (see Plate 15). While again the soldier was stripped of clothing from the waist down and a mirror included with

8 *Philadelphia Photographer*, quoted in Davis, p. 160. Terence Pitts provided a sound account of Bell's career in his MA dissertation, 'William Bell: Philadelphia Photographer' (University of Arizona, 1987), available through Dissertation Abstracts. Many of Bell's medical images, printed in volumes of *Photographs of Special Cases and Specimens* (1865) as issued by the Surgeon General, are now available for study in digital form at http://www.medicalheritage.org/2012/07/digital-highlight-civil-war-photography-from-the-army-medical-museum.

the intention of exposing the chosen treatment as completely as possible, the results are mixed: the mirror reflection of the wound is shadowed and obscured by the crutch, and there would be few viewers capable of ignoring the intense discomfort – doubtless intensified by his enforced immodesty – expressed in the subject's youthful face. Roland Barthes famously advocated 'writing degree zero' in contrast to writing that purported to be 'realistic' but was in fact the product of extreme artifice.[9] The Civil War medical photographs could be described as 'photography degree zero.' One image, taken by an unidentified photographer, presents, close-up and without comment, a pile of amputated limbs awaiting burial.

* * *

The activities of Russell, Barnard, Gardner, and Bell – and of others like them – resulted in the accumulation of thousands of images from the war zone: personnel, both top brass and ordinary soldiers; ordnance; fortifications; maps; feats of engineering; hospitals and the wounded; systems of transport. There are pictures of make-shift bridges, the palisade-like defences built by the Confederates around Atlanta, the ruins of Richmond, field post offices, Southern plantation homes billeted by Union troops, the means of sabotaging railroad lines, and much else. Also, given the complexity of modern warfare as it was developing during the conflict, and changing public attitudes towards the war, the photographers fortunately realised that there were yet other aspects that were just as important to document as anything 'purely' military. An album of 'Scenes of Camp Life – Army of the Potomac' survives, and among its 'scenes' are a soldier's wife and children, doing the laundry, an embalmer seemingly at work on a corpse, two seated lieutenants leaning towards each other as if to stress their comradeship, and, perhaps inevitably, the photographer's own signposted tent.[10] The Sanitary Commission, which raised funds directly from the public to supplement the medical facilities provided by the government, did brisk business in the sale of photographs at its 'fairs,' not just the autographed portraits of prominent generals, but *cartes de visit* scenes its own organisation had made possible, such as shots of the ambulance corps and of smartly uniformed nurses tending the injured. The war increased *consciousness* of photography.

9   Roland Barthes, *Writing Degree Zero* (1953), trans. Annette Lavers and Colin Smith (London: Cape, 1967).
10   There is a page from 'Scenes of Camp Life'" reproduced in Panzer, *Brady*, p. 106, and images from it are scattered through Ward, *The Civil War*.

Indeed, it could be argued that the pervasiveness of the medium during the conflict helped produce a photographic 'way of seeing.' It is instructive that things that really occurred but which could not actually be photographed *as* they happened – such as an amputation – were deliberately re-staged for the camera. The poet Walt Whitman – who would later pretend to grumble to Horace Traubel that he had been 'photographed, photographed, photographed, until the very cameras themselves were tired' of him – was particularly aware of the medium's omnivorous and democratic properties. He titled a gathering of his Civil War prose sketches 'City Photographs,' and often his poems were built upon a series of exact partial impressions.[11] In the short poem 'Cavalry Crossing a Ford,' for example, with its 'Behold the brown-faced men, each group, each person, a picture,' the troops, as they ride into a stream, are presented as if individually framed by a camera. They are 'brown-faced' because burnt by the wind or sun but possibly also because they are each seen *as* 'a picture,' most likely a sepia-toned *carte de visit*.

Timothy H. O'Sullivan – who at the onset of hostilities worked for Brady before being lured away by Gardner – was the most artistically gifted of the Civil War photographers. (He would later produce sublime landscapes of the West for both the King and the Wheeler surveys.) Many of his images suggest meanings beyond those merely denoted by their subject matter. In a series of views of Ulysses S. Grant meeting with his generals near the Massaponax Baptist Church, Virginia, on May 21, 1864, just after the Battle of Spotsylvania Courthouse, he managed to convey a sense of the importance of a particular moment as time passes (see Plate 16). By all accounts, the meeting was more of a post mortem on the preceding engagement than preparation for the next, but in the picture battle plans seem to be in the making. In order to achieve a 'military prospect' for plans, it was routine to elevate the camera. Here O'Sullivan was able to do it drastically by shooting from an upper-storey window of the church. We look down on the scene in the round, the officers seated at long pews taken from the church, as if at a stage, but because the actors appear unaware of our presence we become silent witnesses to the drama.[12]

---

11   Horace Traubel, *With Walt Whitman in Camden*, vol. 1 (orig. 1906; New York: Roman and Littlefield, 1961), p. 367. For Whitman and photography, see Ed Folsom, *Whitman's Native Representations* (Cambridge and New York: Cambridge University Press, 1994), and for commentary on the Civil War as a crucible fusing Whitman and photgraphy, see Timothy Sweet, *Traces of War: Poetry, Photography, and the Crisis of the Union* (Baltimore and London: Johns Hopkins University Press, 1990).

12   For more on O'Sullivan in the Civil War, the extensive data in James

* * *

Civil War photographs – especially when scanned first-hand, as it were, as tintypes, as stereocards, as separate collodian prints or collected in the pages of limited-circulation books such as Barnard's or Gardner's – made a profound impression in their own time. Many of them received broad circulation in engraved form in such illustrated magazines as *Harper's* and *Frank Leslie's Weekly*. A reporter for the New York *Evening Post*, after a visit to see the war views exhibited at Brady's gallery in the city in 1866, wrote that they illustrated 'the prominent incidents of the war with remarkable fidelity.' 'The military camps, fortifications, reviews, siege trains,' he continued, 'the farmhouses, plantations and famous buildings of the south – the groups of [...] officers in the field and on the decks of of our war vessels – the horrors of war, and its higher aspects as seen around the bivouac fires, and all portrayed exactly as they were, as no pen could describe them.'[13]

In particular, images of what the writer for the *Evening Post* called 'the horrors of war' always made the greatest impact. Barely a month after the Maryland battle of Antietam in 1862, a journalist for the *New York Times* wrote up his impressions of pictures of the Antietam dead displayed at Brady's premises (see Plate 17): 'We recognize the battle-field as a reality, but it stands as a remote one. It is like a funeral next door [...] But it is very different when the hearse stops at your own door, and the corpse is carried out over your own threshold.' 'Mr. Brady,' the reporter continued, 'has done something to bring home to us the terrible reality and earnestness of war. If he has not brought bodies and laid them in our dooryards and along streets, he has done something very like it.' The effect of such images was both general and individual. Generally, they were symbolic: their early viewers could not evade the knowledge that in one day (September 17, 1862) at Antietam, 26,000 died – and, with the passing of time, that day has 'achieved immortality,' as the photo-historian William Frassanito put it, 'as the bloodiest single day in the history of the United States.'[14]

D. Horan, *Timothy O'Sullivan: America's Forgotten Photographer* (Garden City, NY: Doubleday, 1966) should be supplemented and corrected by commentary in the works cited above by Frassanito, Davis, and Trachtenberg.

13   For more on the transmission of the war photographs, see Michael L. Carlebach, *The Origins of Photojournalism in America* (Washington, DC, and London: Smithsonian Institution Press, 1992), especially pp. 62–101. Report in New York *Evening Post*, reprinted in Panzer, *Brady*, p. 221.

14   *New York Times*, October 20, 1862, excerpted at length elsewhere in this book;

The reporter for the *New York Times* pointed to their effect on individuals: 'These pictures have a terrible distinctness.' 'By the aid of a magnifying-glass,' he observed, 'the very features of the slain may be distinguished. We would scarce choose to be in the gallery when one of the women bending over them should recognize a husband, a son, or a brother in the still, lifeless lines of bodies that lie ready for the gaping trenches.'[15] This belief that the realism of the photographs of the dead offered a sense of at least potential recognition was very prevalent. We see it at work in the response to such images by Oliver Wendell Holmes, Harvard medical professor, man of letters, and amateur photographer, who was sent Antietam pictures in stereocard form.

When Holmes looked at them, most likely with the 3D effect gained by using the stereoviewer he had invented, they brought back memories of his desperate search for his son, a captain on the Union side, a few months earlier, when he feared – mistakenly, as it turned out – that the young man had been seriously wounded in the battle. Readers of his *Atlantic Monthly* column, in which he had earlier described the battlefield 'hunt for the captain,' would have been aware that his comments on the Antietam views had a personal edge:

> It was so nearly like visiting the battlefield to look over these views, that all the emotions excited by the actual sight of the sordid scene, strewed with rags and wrecks, came back to us, and we buried them in the recesses of our cabinet as we would have buried the mutilated remains of the dead they too vividly represented.[16]

* * *

Such images as those of the Antietam dead – if not immediately 'buried' – demanded a second look, and it was likely to be more painful than the first. When they were published as engravings in *Harper's Weekly* the writer who introduced them also talked – and in an instructive manner – of his compulsion to examine the originals with a magnifying glass: 'Minute as are

---

also quoted in Frassanito, *Antietam*, pp. 15–17, with Frassanito's comment on p. 17.
15   *New York Times*, October 20, 1862, excerpted at length elsewhere in this book; also in Susan Sontag, *Regarding the Pain of Others* (New York: Picador, 2003), pp. 62–63, where it features in a probing consideration of the ethics of looking. Frassanito, in *Antietam*, has actually identified some of the dead, and researched their brief life stories.
16   Oliver Wendell Holmes, 'Doings of the Sunbeam,' *Atlantic Monthly* (1863), quoted in Sweet, p. 119.

the features of the dead, and unrecognisable by the naked eye, you can, by bringing a magnifying glass to bear on them, identify not merely the general outline, but actual expression.' In such seeking after 'expression' in these war pictures there was, of course, a desire to make sense of the carnage, a desire for meaning. We can sometimes see that desire at work in the titles, captions and legends that the photographic entrepreneurs and photographers affixed to the images. Brady, in presenting a particular view of corpses at Antietam (probably taken by Gardner), found a purely mechanistic explanation: 'The bodies of the dead [...] strewn thickly beside the fence [...] shows that the fighting was severe at this point on [that] bloody day.'[17]

O'Sullivan, in titling a picture of the dead taken after the battle of Gettysburg in 1863 – perhaps his best-known work – opted for a pastoral metaphor: 'A Harvest of Death' (see Plate 18). Gettysburg proved to be the point at which the war had turned in favour of the North, so in retrospect it might well have seemed 'natural' that such sacrifice of life had been required to achieve it. In the photograph, the bloated bodies are strewn across a field as a kind of substitute for the wheat or barley that would normally have grown there. When Gardner wrote his commentary for this image at its incorporation into his *Sketch Book* he went further: he identified the fallen troops as Confederates 'killed in the frantic efforts to break the steady lines of an army of patriots, whose heroism only excelled theirs in motive, they paid with life the price of their treason.' He then added: 'Such a picture conveys a useful moral: It shows the blank horror and reality of war, in opposition to its pageantry. Here are the dreadful details! Let them aid in preventing another such calamity falling upon the nation.'[18]

All too often 'the dreadful details' were exactly what they seemed, and the photographs did present what Gardner aptly termed 'the blank horror' of war. People were shocked by depictions of what could not be naturalised, such as the confusion of the living and the dead in field hospitals, of ghastly piles of amputated limbs outside them, and of the dead – either unburied or as skeletal remains – being disinterred for re-burial some place else. Whitman had written about such sights, and now here they were in newspaper illustrations, engraved from photographs. And the Northern public was angered by the photographs of suvivors of the South's notorious Andersonville prisoner of war camp. These pages of starved and emaciated victims in *Frank Leslie's Weekly* and other journals, many with untreated wounds, constitute some of the earliest atrocity photographs, and as yet there was no vocabulary to deal with them. True, they

17   *Harper's Weekly* 6 (October 18, 1862), quoted in Davis, p. 152. One of Brady's lecture notes, as quoted by Trachtenberg, p. 86.
18   Gardner, *Sketch Book* reprint, legend to plate 36 of vol. 1.

led to calls for vengeance for 'rebel cruelties,' but the concept of photographs providing evidence of crimes against humanity – crimes greater, that is, than war itself – was yet to arise.[19]

Sometimes 'the dreadful details' were not what they seemed. Compare two images taken by Gardner on the Gettysburg battlefield and included in his *Sketch Book*, 'A Sharpshooter's Last Sleep' (see Plate 19) and 'Home of a Rebel Sharpshooter.' Despite their captions – which in the case of the first claims the man was 'lying as he fell [...] [his] cap and gun [...] evidently thrown behind him by the violence of the shock' and which in the second says the photographer had 'found in a lonely place the covert of a rebel sharpshooter, and photographed the scene presented here' – the images depict the *same* man in not quite the same place. As Frassanito observed, for one or other of these pictures, or for both, the body and other things, notably the rifle, *must* have been moved for the photograph.[20]

But it would be a mistake to think of the fabrication of such images as the most important thing about them. Note the naturalizing title Gardner gave to 'A Sharpshooter's Last Sleep' and the sense of *order* in the image: the line of the rifle, the cap near to its owner's head, angled as if it had just been taken off, all captured from a lowered height that makes the rocks protectively surround this outpost. The *New York Times* reviewer, although not speaking of this particular image, was again perceptive in finding 'poetry' in such views of the dead: 'There is a poetry in the scene, that no green fields or smiling landscapes can possess. Here lie men who have not hesitated to seal and stamp their convictions with their blood – men who have flung themselves into the great gulf of the unknown to teach the world that there are truths dearer than life.' Here we have fabriction – art, actually – in the service of consolation. 'Have heart, poor mother,' the *Times* writer continued, in an extended peroration that offered in words the solace that *no* photograph ever could provide.[21] Nevertheless, the key feature of these Civil War images – whether examples of photography degree zero or marked by visual devices that might more readily be associated with painting and drawing – is that they both record aspects of the national tragedy and at least intimate ways in which it might be understood.

19   For discussion of such matters, see Geoffrey Batchen, Mick Gidley, Nancy Miller, and Jay Prosser, eds, *Picturing Atrocity: Photography in Crisis* (London: Reaktion, 2012).

20   Gardner, *Sketch Book* reprint, legends to plates 40 and 41 of vol. 1. Frassanito's discussion, more complex than my summary and part-crediting O'Sullivan for these images, is in *Gettysburg*, pp. 186–95.

21   *New York Times*, October 20, 1862, excerpted below.

Mathew Brady's Photographs:

Pictures of the Dead at Antietam

The following is excerpted from the *New York Times*, October 20, 1862, p. 5. It is a report, by an unidentified writer, of a visit during the Civil War to Mathew B. Brady's Manhattan gallery and studio. Brady (1823?–1896), the leading American portrait photographer of his generation, and the most prominent photographic entrepreneur of the time, was exhibiting recently made battlefield views taken by employees and associates he had sent into the field. In 1862 the medium was not yet 25 years old, and the reporter probably lacked much personal familiarity with it – at one point speaking of it capturing likenesses on 'canvas,' as if the images were paintings. But he (or possibly she) gives a very accurate description of what was on show in the gallery, provides a sense of the wartime impact of the photographs and is remarkably perceptive.

The living that throng Broadway care little perhaps for the Dead at Antietam, but we fancy they would jostle less carelessly down the great thoroughfare, saunter less at their ease, were a few dripping bodies, fresh from the field, laid along the pavement. There would be a gathering up of skirts and a careful picking of way; conversation would be less lively, and the general air of pedestrians more subdued. As it is, the dead of the battlefield come to us very rarely, even in dreams. We see the list in the morning paper at breakfast but dismiss its recollection with coffee. There is a confused mass of names, but they are all strangers; we forget the horrible significance that dwells amid the jumble of type. The roll we read is being called over in Eternity, and pale, trembling lips are answering to it. Shadowy fingers point from the page to a field where even imagination is loth to follow. Each of these little names that the printer struck off so lightly last night, whistling over his work, and that we speak with a clip of the tongue, represents a bleeding, mangled corpse. It is a thunderbolt that will crash into some brain – a dull, dead, remorseless weight that will fall upon some heart, straining it to breaking. There is nothing very terrible to us, however, in the list, though our sensations might be different if the newspaper carrier left the names on the battle-field and the bodies at our doors instead.

We recognize the battle-field as a reality, but it stands as a remote one. It is like a funeral next door. The crape on the bell-pull tells there is death in the house, and in the close carriage that rolls away with muffled wheels you know there rides a woman to whom the world is very dark now. But you only see the mourners in the last of the long line of carriages – they ride very jollily and at their ease, smoking cigars in a furtive and discursive manner, perhaps, and were it not for the black gloves they wear, which the deceased was wise and liberal enough to furnish, it might be a wedding for all the world would know. It attracts your attention, but does not enlist your sympathy. But it is very different when the hearse stops at your own door, and the corpse is carried out over your own threshold – you know whether it is a wedding or a funeral then, without looking at the color of the gloves worn. Those who lose friends in battle know what battle-fields are, and our Marylanders, with their door-yards strewed with the dead and dying, and their houses turned into hospitals for the wounded, know what battle-fields are.

Mr. BRADY has done something to bring home to us the terrible reality and earnestness of war. If he has not brought bodies and laid them in our dooryards and along streets, he has done something very like it. At the door of his gallery hangs a little placard, 'The Dead of Antietam.' Crowds of people are constantly going up the stairs; follow them, and you find them bending over photographic views of that fearful battle-field, taken immediately after the action. Of all objects of horror one would think the battle-field should stand pre-eminent, that it should bear away the palm of repulsiveness. But, on the contrary, there is a terrible fascination about it that draws one near these pictures, and makes him loth to leave them. You will see hushed, reverend groups standing around these weird copies of carnage, bending down to look in the pale faces of the dead, chained by the strange spell that dwells in dead men's eyes. It seems somewhat singular that the same sun that looked down on the faces of the slain, blistering them, blotting out from the bodies all semblance to humanity, and hastening corruption, should thus have caught their features upon canvas, and given them perpetuity for ever. But so it is.

These poor subjects could not give the sun sittings, and they are taken as they fell, their poor hands clutching the grass around them in spasms of pain, or reaching out for help which none gave. Union soldier and Confederate, side by side, here they lie, the red light of battle faded from their eyes [...] The ground whereon they lie is torn by shot and shell, the grass is trampled down by tread of hot, hurrying feet, and little rivulets that can scarcely be water are trickling along the earth like tears over a mother's face. It is a bleak, barren plain [...] But there is a poetry in the scene, that no green fields or smiling landscapes can possess. Here lie men who have not hesitated to seal and stamp their convictions with their blood – men who have flung themselves into the great gulf of the unknown to teach the world that there are truths dearer than life, wrongs and shames more to be dreaded than death [...].

There is one side of the picture that the sun did not catch, one phase that has escaped photographic skill. It is the background of widows and orphans, torn from the bosom of their natural protectors by the red remorseless hand of Battle [...] Homes have been made desolate, and the light of life in thousands of hearts has been quenched forever. All this desolation imagination must paint – broken hearts cannot be photographed.

These pictures have a terrible distinctness. By the aid of a magnifying-glass the very features of the slain may be distinguished. We would scarce choose to be in the gallery when one of the women bending over them should recognize a husband, a son, or a brother in the still, lifeless lines of bodies that lie ready for the gaping trenches. For these trenches have a terror for a woman's heart, that goes far to outweigh all others that hover over the battle-field. How can a mother bear to know that the boy, whose slumbers she has cradled, and whose head her bosom pillowed until the rolling drums called him forth – whose poor, pale face, could she reach it, should find the same pillow again [...] when, but for the privelege of touching that corpse, of kissing once more the lips though white and cold, of smoothing back the hair from the brow and cleansing it of blood stains, she would give all the remaining years of life that Heaven has allotted her – how can this mother bear to know that in a shallow trench, hastily dug, rude hands have thrown him. She would have handled the poor corpse so tenderly, have prized the boon of caring for it so dearly – yet, even the imperative office of hiding the dead from sight has been done by those who thought it trouble, and were only glad when their work ended.

Have heart, poor mother, grieve not without hope, mourn not without consolation. This is not the last of your boy [...] there is reserved for him a crown only heroes and martyrs are permitted to wear.

AMPUTATIONS AND PROSTHETIC LIMBS

'The Invalid Corps' (song)

It is estimated that some 60,000 lost limbs in the Civil War, so many that the US government established the 'Great Civil War Benefaction' to provide prosthetic limbs for victims. In 1863 the Invalid Corps was established in the Union army, renamed in 1864 the Veteran Research Corps. A popular song with the title 'The Invalid Corps' from the same period focuses on an unsuccessful volunteer who fails his medical examination and then serves with the Invalids.

The Invalid Corps

I wanted much to go to war,
And went to be examined;
The surgeon looked me o'er and o'er,
My back and chest he hammered.
Said he, 'You're not the man for me,
Your lungs are much affected,
And likewise both your eyes are cock'd,
And otherwise defected.'

> **CHORUS**
> So, now I'm with the Invalids,
> And cannot go and fight, sir!
> The doctor told me so, you know,
> Of course it must be right, sir!

While I was there a host of chaps
For reasons were exempted,
Old 'pursy,' he was laid aside,
To pass he had attempted.
The doctor said, 'I do not like

Your corporosity, sir!
You'll "breed a famine" in the camp
Wherever you might be, sir!'

CHORUS

There came a fellow, mighty tall,
A 'knock-kneed overgrowner,'
The Doctor said, 'I ain't got time
To take and look you over.'
Next came along a little chap,
Who was 'bout two foot nothing,
The Doctor said, 'You'd better go
And tell your marm you're coming!'

CHORUS

Some had the ticerdolerreou,
Some what they call 'brown critters,'
And some were 'lank and lazy' too,
Some were too 'fond of bitters.'
Some had 'cork legs' and some 'one eye,'
With backs deformed and crooked,
I'll bet you'd laugh'd till you had cried,
To see how 'cute' they looked.

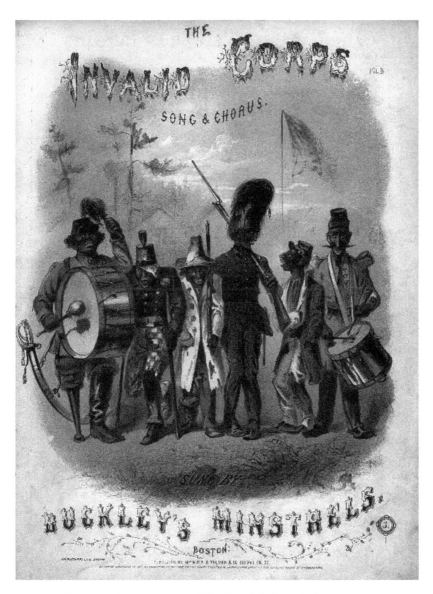

Figure 8: Front cover to 'The Invalid Corps' sheet music

The Case of Napoleon Perkins

Dillon Jackson Carroll (University of Georgia)

The most vivid memory Napoleon Perkins could still remember from the Battle of Chancellorsville was the 'limbs, leaves, and blossoms' of the apple trees 'falling in all directions' around him. It was May 3, 1863. The 5th Maine Battery, Perkins' battery, had just unlimbered in an apple orchard on the battlefield and began firing canister into the Confederate infantry. Rebel artillery responded in kind, opening fire upon Perkins and his 5th Maine comrades. All around him, apple blossoms fell from the attack. Of course, the apple blossoms were not the sole casualties, and members of the 5th Maine were struck and 'falling at the guns.' The 'schrieks [sic] & groans' of the wounded men were 'heartrending' and something Perkins never forgot. When a horse was wounded, Perkins dashed up to unhitch the creature and replace it with a spare horse. But as he was undoing the hitch, a Minié ball slammed into his right leg, just above the knee.[1]

While Perkins did not immediately know it, his injury would eventually result in an amputation of his leg. He became one of an estimated 60,000 Civil War soldiers who lost a limb in the war, one of an estimated 45,000 to survive the operation, a macabre fraternity of sorts. In his old age at the turn of the century, Perkins' children prevailed upon him to write a memoir. Perkins' memoir is unique because we know so little about the lives of Civil War amputees after they limped home. His writing gives historians insight into the physical and emotional anguish amputees endured as they struggled to rebuild themselves into men.[2]

1   Napoleon B. Perkins, *The Memoirs of N.B. Perkins* (Concord, NH: New Hampshire Historical Society, unpublished), p. 10.
2   Laurann Figg and Jane Farrell-Beck, 'Amputation in the Civil War: Physical

Back on the battlefield, rescue came in the form of comrades, who brought a stretcher, lifted Perkins, and carried him away from the fight. They set him down about three miles from the battlefield, at an old plantation house, now serving as a makeshift hospital. He spent a long sleepless night in that house, which was 'full of wounded men,' some of them 'mortally wounded and dying' while others were delirious. 'Some were groaning, others were praying, while others were singing, while still others were swearing,' Perkins remembered. 'I shall never forget that night and have often dreamed of it.' Perkins may have suffered with post-traumatic stress disorder, considering a signal symptom of PTSD was re-experiencing a traumatic memory through dreams, flashbacks, or hallucinations. Perkins indicated as much, acknowledging his long night in the field hospital had haunted his dreams years after the war.[3]

The next day, Perkins was removed from the field hospital, and endured a long and painful trip to St. Aloysius Hospital, in Washington, DC. Once there, Perkins hoped his leg would heal, but after several weeks his leg remained inflamed and swollen. Then slowly it began to mortify and turn forebodingly black. Likely, a streptococcal bacterium had infected the wound in his leg and was devastating the tissue. By the end of May, surgeons at St. Aloysius told Perkins that his 'leg must come off' or he would not 'live three days longer.' His leg was amputated the next day. He was semi-conscious during the operation, because the surgeon was afraid to give him too much ether anesthetic.[4]

Walt Whitman believed that it was the wounded who endured the war's 'fearfulest test.' In many ways he was right. Wounded soldiers recovering from injury were expected to embody a patriotic endurance. Though they were in intense pain, they were expected to never complain, and instead be cheerful. It was through this example that they could serve as inspirations to all those around them. Female nurses were the enforcers of this behavior. While roaming the ward of a hospital in Georgia, Kate Cumming lamented that 'none of the glories of war were presented' in the hospital. But, she wrote, 'if

and Social Dimensions,' *Journal of the History of Medicine and Allied Sciences* 48 (1993), pp. 456–63; Megan Kate Nelson, 'Napoleon Perkins Loses His Leg,' *New York Times*, May 29, 2013; Megan Kate Nelson, *Ruin Nation: Destruction and the American Civil War* (Athens, GA: University of Georgia Press, 2012).

3 Perkins, *Memoirs of N.B. Perkins*, p. 12; Eric T. Dean, Jr., *Shook Over Hell: Post-Traumatic Stress, Vietnam and the Civil War* (Cambridge, MA: Harvard University Press, 1997), p. 127.

4 Perkins, *Memoirs of N.B. Perkins*, p. 12; Margaret Humphreys, *Marrow of Tragedy: The Health Crisis of the American Civil War* (Baltimore: Johns Hopkins University Press, 2013), pp. 31–34.

uncomplaining endurance is glory, we had plenty of it.' While at St. Aloysius, Napoleon befriended a fellow amputee named John Erway. John Erway had lost his leg below the knee, but 'he was a jolly good fellow and at times did not seem to mind the loss of his leg.' However, when the sun went down, the nurses went to bed, and the halls grew dark, Erway's anxiety spilled out. His disability was going to change his entire life, and he knew it. 'After getting acquainted with [Erway], I could see how much he felt the loss as he told me once it would change the whole course of his life,' Perkins wrote. This became the script for many amputees following their injury. They were never allowed to complain, and instead, were expected to persevere, with optimistic fortitude.[5]

Amputation threatened to emasculate men. First, men worried about how they would be viewed in the eyes of the opposite sex. Walter Lenoir was wounded at the Battle of Ox Hill, and as he lay writhing in the dirt, his mind wandered to things his disability would deprive him of. 'First I thought of my favorite sport of trout fishing, which I would have to give up. Then I thought of skating, swimming, and partridge hunting,' Lenoir wrote. 'Before all these things I thought sadly of women; for I was not old enough to have given up the thought of women.' Because of the initial helpless condition of the wounded, many female nurses compared amputees to children, infantilizing them. While working as a nurse in Washington, Louisa May Alcott daily washed the prostrated men in her ward, remembering: '[S]ome of them took the performance like sleepy children, leaning their tired heads against me as I worked.' When over 50 soldiers arrived at Hannah Ropes' ward, she wrote: '[T] hey sank upon us to care for them [...] helpless as babes.' Confederate nurse Ada Bacot scribbled in her diary: 'It is sad to think of the hundreds of disabled men this war is producing, many will be of no possible use them selves or of any one else.'[6]

5   Perkins, *The Memoirs of N.B. Perkins*, p. 16; Frances M. Clarke, *War Stories: Suffering and Sacrifice in the Civil War North* (Chicago: University of Chicago Press, 2011), pp. 8–15; Drew Gilpin Faust, *This Republic of Suffering: Death and the American Civil War* (New York: Knopf, 2008), pp. 10–31.

6   Walter Lenoir diary, Lenoir Family Papers, Southern Historical Collection, Chapel Hill, University of North Carolina, p. 23; Bessie Z. Jones, ed., *Hospital Sketches by Louisa May Alcott* (Cambridge, MA: Harvard University Press, 1960), pp. 29–31; John R. Brumgardt, ed., *Civil War Nurse: The Diary and Letters of Hannah Ropes* (Knoxville, TN: University of Tennessee Press, 1980), p. 53; Jean V. Berlin, ed., *A Confederate Nurse: The Diary of Ada W. Bacot* (Columbia, SC: University of South Carolina Press, 1994), p. 140; James Marten, *Sing Not War: The Lives of Union and Confederate Veterans in the Gilded Age* (Chapel Hill, NC:

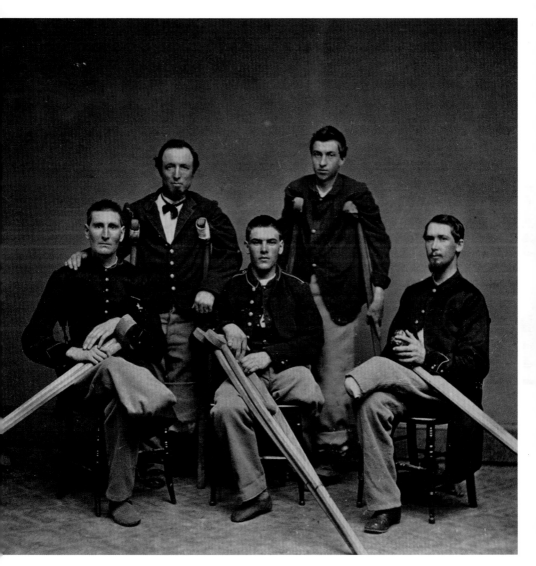

Plate 1: Civil War veterans (courtesy National Library of Medicine).

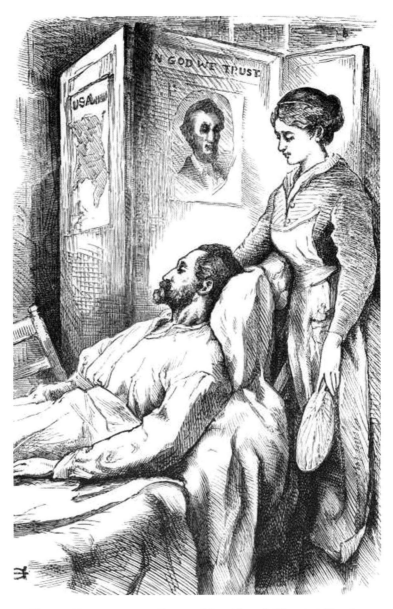

Plate 2: Frontispiece to Louisa May Alcott's *Hospital Sketches* (1869).

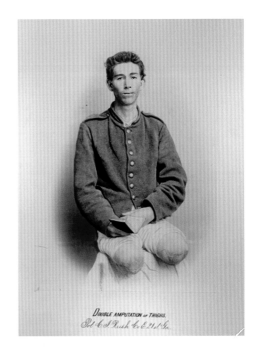

Plates 3 and 4: Columbus J. Rush, Private, Co. E, 21st Georgia Volunteers. Amputation of both thighs following shell wounds received at Fort Steadman, Virginia, March 25, 1865. Image reproduced courtesy of the Otis Collection, National Museum of Health and Medicine, Maryland.

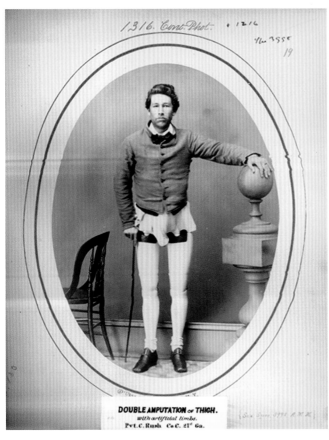

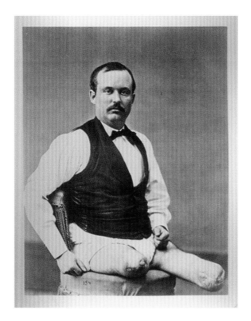

Plates 5 and 6: Corporal Charles N. Lapham, 1st Vermont Cavalry. Amputation following wounds from solid shot near Boonsborough, Maryland, July 8, 1863. Image reproduced courtesy of the Otis Collection, National Museum of Health and Medicine, Maryland.

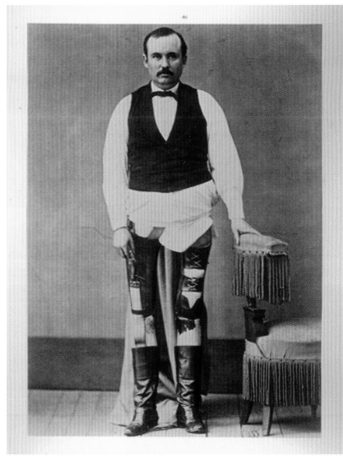

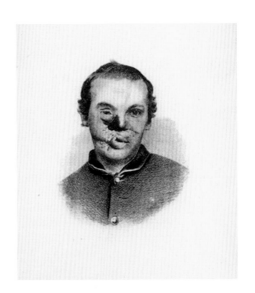

Plates 7 and 8: Carlton Burgan, Private, Co. B, Permall Legion, Maryland Volunteers. Case of osteonecrosis of the jaw subsequent to mercury overdose. Image reproduced courtesy of the Otis Collection, National Museum of Health and Medicine, Maryland.

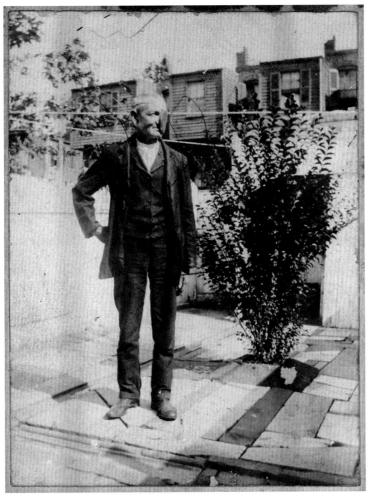

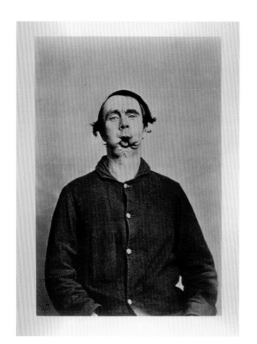

Plates 9 and 10: Private Rowland Ward, Co. E, 4th New York Heavy Artillery. Cheiloplasty following shell damage to jaw at Ream's Station, Virginia, August 25, 1864. Image reproduced by courtesy of the Otis Collection, National Museum of Health and Medicine, Maryland.

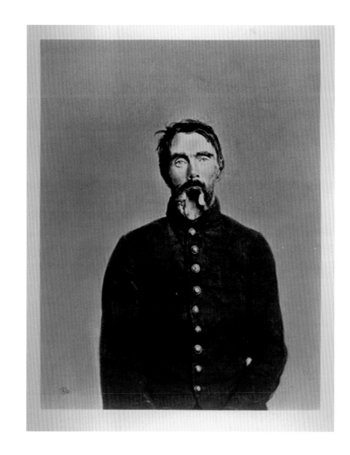

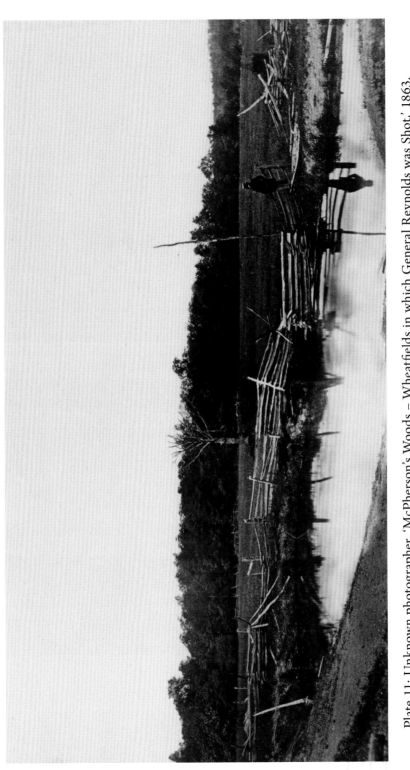

Plate 11: Unknown photographer, 'McPherson's Woods – Wheatfields in which General Reynolds was Shot,' 1863. Digital scan of albumen print. Courtesy Library of Congress.

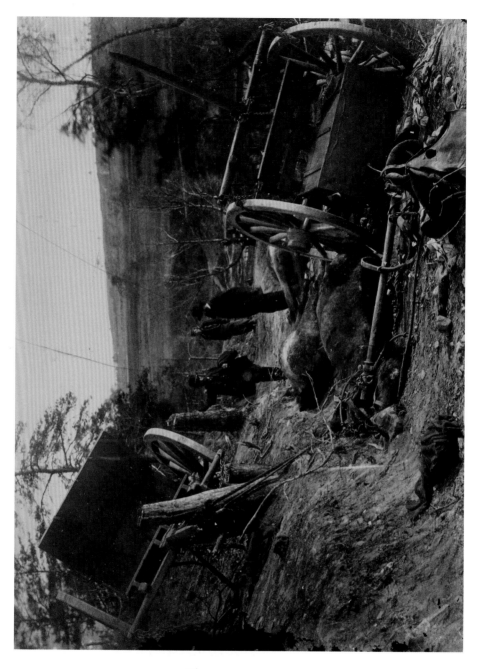

Plate 12: Andrew J. Russell, 'Rebel Caisson Destroyed by Federal Shells at Fredricksburg, 3 May, 1863.' Digital scan of albumen print. Courtesy Library of Congress.

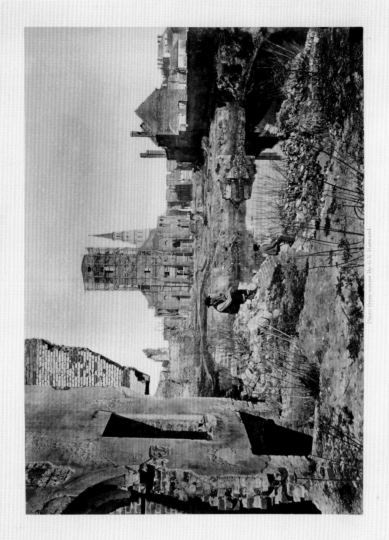

RUINS IN CHARLESTON, S.C.

Photo from nature by G.N. Barnard

Plate 13: George N. Barnard, 'Ruins at Charleston, SC,', 1864. Digital scan of albumen print from Barnard's *Photographic Views*, 1866. Courtesy George Eastman House International Museum of Photography and Film.

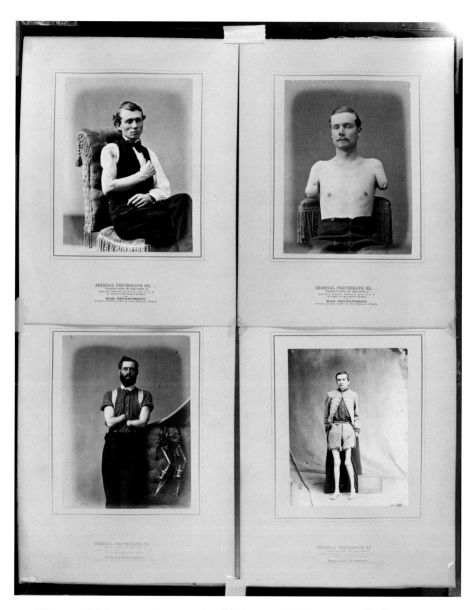

Plate 14: Unknown photographer(s), 'Surgical photographs [...] prepared under supervision of [...] War Dept., Surgeon General's Office, Army Medical Museum,' c. 1866. Digital scan of album plates. Courtesy Library of Congress.

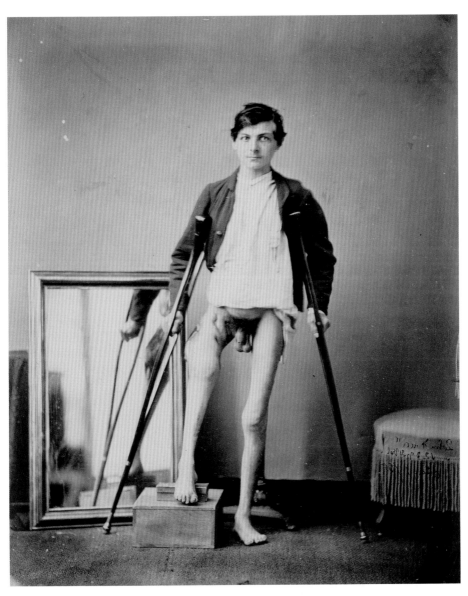

Plate 15: Willam H. Bell, 'Gunshot Fracture of the Shaft of the Right Femur, United with Great Shortening and Deformity,' 1865. Digital scan of albumen silver print. Courtesy J. Paul Getty Museum.

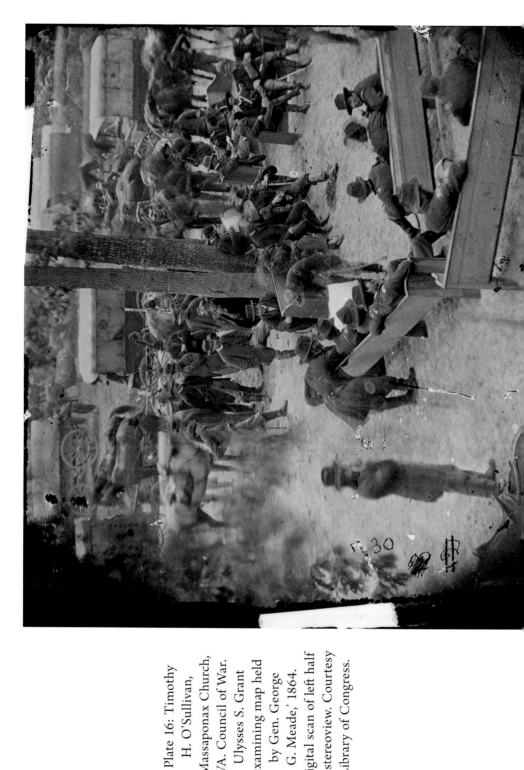

Plate 16: Timothy H. O'Sullivan, 'Massaponax Church, VA. Council of War. Ulysses S. Grant examining map held by Gen. George G. Meade,' 1864. Digital scan of left half of stereoview. Courtesy Library of Congress.

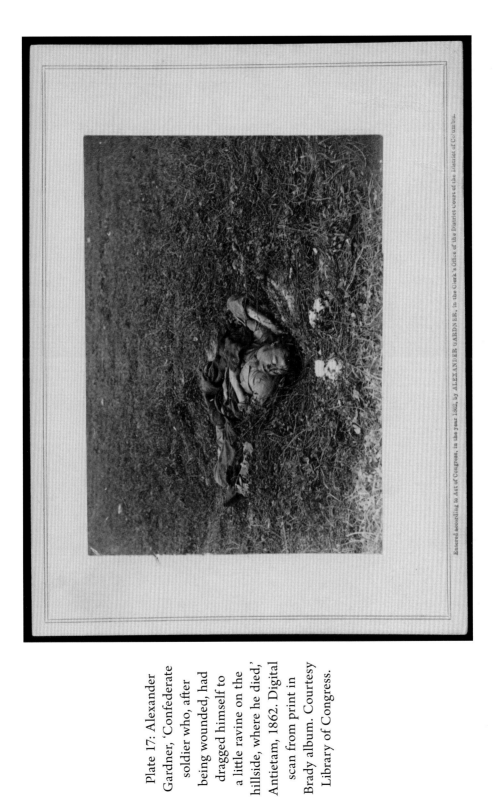

Entered according to Act of Congress, in the year 1862, by ALEXANDER GARDNER, in the Clerk's Office of the District Court of the District of Columbia.

Plate 17: Alexander Gardner, 'Confederate soldier who, after being wounded, had dragged himself to a little ravine on the hillside, where he died,' Antietam, 1862. Digital scan from print in Brady album. Courtesy Library of Congress.

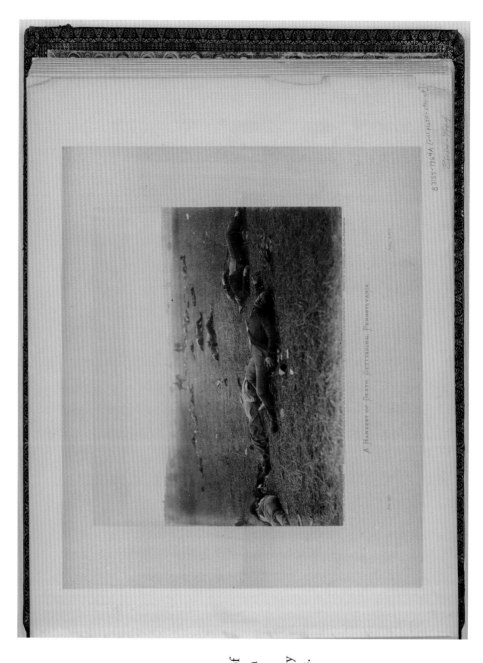

Plate 18: Timothy H. O'Sullivan, 'A Harvest of Death,' 1863. Digital scan of albumen print from Gardner's *Sketch Book*, 1866. Courtesy Library of Congress.

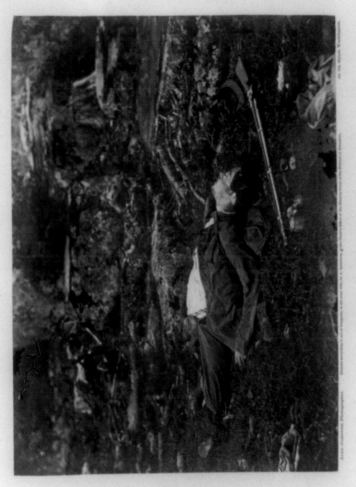

Plate 19: Alexander Gardner, 'A Sharpshooter's Last Sleep,' 1863. Black and white digital scan of print from Gardner's *Sketch Book*, 1866. Courtesy Library of Congress.

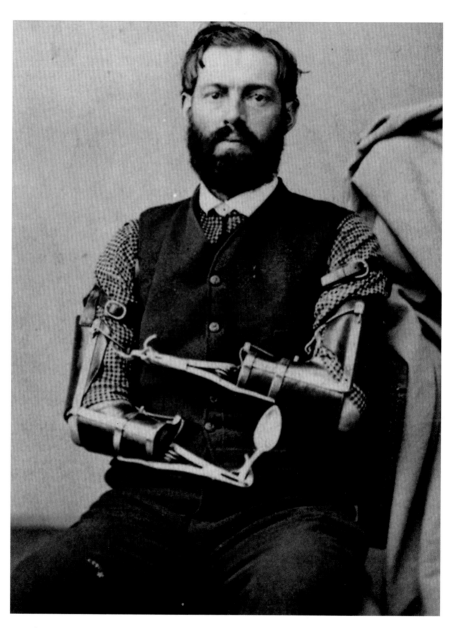

Plate 20: Samuel Decker, Union veteran, at the Army Medical Museum
(1867).

Mobility was step one on the road to manhood. Most amputees turned to prosthetic limbs. The Civil War was a boon for the prosthetic limb industry. Between 1845 and 1861, 34 patents were issued for prosthetic limbs. Between 1861 and 1873, 133 patents were issued. Prosthetics were important for mobility, but also they were important for amputees to become conspicuous in civilian society. 'At an age when appearances are reality,' wrote Oliver Wendell Holmes, 'it becomes important to provide the cripple with a limb which shall be presentable in polite society, where misfortunes of a certain obtrusiveness may be pitied, but are never tolerated under the chandeliers.' In 1864, Perkins was transferred to Stanton Hospital, and while there he was measured and fitted for a Jewett leg, a high-caliber prosthetic limb. When he first strapped into his Jewett leg, he was 'expecting to be able to walk at once' but was disappointed that he 'could hardly walk with the aid of my crutches.' He returned to his cot 'feeling rather blue' but not defeated. After repeated tries, Perkins finally learned to walk without aid on his prosthetic limb. 'Shall always remember the first step I took without help,' he wrote. 'Felt as proud as a little child learning to walk.'[7]

Napoleon Perkins was honorably discharged in 1864 – his army days were done. He returned to civilian society with a wooden leg and very few prospects. In addition, he felt overwhelmed with embarrassment over his disability. He probably never read the advice from the editor of *The Cripple*, a hospital newspaper: 'Do not vex yourself with thoughts of inferiority,' wrote the editor to disabled readers, 'banish them by finding something to do or say worthwhile.' But Perkins had difficulty banishing thoughts of inferiority, a difficulty that lasted throughout his life. 'My crippled condition I felt very keenly,' Perkins wrote, 'and as for that matter, I never entirely got past that feeling.' Moving in with his sister and her husband in Lebanon, New Hampshire, Perkins enrolled in school to continue his education.[8]

University of North Carolina Press, 2011), p. 56; Brian Craig Miller, in Stephen Berry, ed., *Weirding the War: Stories from the Civil War's Ragged Edges* (Athens, GA: University of Georgia Press, 2011), pp. 302–5.

7   Laurann Figg and Jane Farrell-Beck, 'Amputation in the Civil War: Physical and Social Dimensions,' *Journal of the History of Medicine and Allied Sciences* 48 (1993), pp. 456–63; Oliver Wendell Holmes, 'The Human Wheel, Its Spokes and Felloes,' *Atlantic Monthly* (1863), p. 574; Katherine Ott, David Serlin, and Stephen Mihm, eds, *Artificial Parts, Practical Lives: Modern Histories of Prosthetics* (New York: New York University Press, 2002); Perkins, *The Memoirs of N.B. Perkins*, p. 20.

8   *The Cripple* (U.S. General Hospital, Alexandria, VA), November 12, 1864; Perkins, *The Memoirs of N.B. Perkins*, p. 25.

But by 1865, his coffers were dry and he was forced to leave school and look for work. He became a 'tramp,' traveling the country far and wide in search of wage work. By 1873, America became aware that it had a 'tramp problem,' as legions of young men traveled in search of work, many of them veterans. 'Why is it that so large a number of the business men throughout the country hesitate to employ the returned soldier?' asked one veteran in a newspaper editorial. 'There is no disguising it boys; the people are afraid of us!' Perkins traveled to East Haverhill, where he briefly worked as a clerk until he was laid off. In 1866, he split time between New Hampshire, Maine, and Boston, looking for work. He felt like he visited every place of employment in Lewiston, but every cotton factory and shoe shop that he applied had owners that 'all seemed to feel sorry' for young Perkins, but 'they had no work that a one leg man could do.' He traveled to Toledo, Ohio, and Detroit, Michigan, and spent time in Montreal, Canada, and Carlisle, Massachusetts; but each locale furnished no one willing to offer him a job. He found plenty of pity, and kind people willing to buy him breakfast, but no steady work. He briefly clerked in Lebanon, before he finally had his big break when he was offered a job in a millinery shop in Groveton, New Hampshire.[9]

It was also in Groveton that he met Jennie Shedd, his future wife. She was a young 17-year-old domestic servant in 1869 when they first met. The two were married several years later. Why did Jennie marry Perkins? We will never know for sure, but perhaps Jennie was attracted to Perkins because he was dependent upon her, reversing the gender roles of the time. She would not have been the only one. 'Dear Richard while I sympathize in your terrible suffering & loss,' wrote Lizinka Ewell to her husband Richard after he had lost his leg, 'it is only womanly to remember that one of its consequences will be to oblige you to remain at home & make me more necessary to you & another is that [...] now I will suit you better than any one else, if only because I will love you better.' Napoleon Perkins wrote that Jennie had been 'a true helpmate [...] waiting upon me and bearing my faults with a cheerfulness that none could excel.'[10]

In Groveton, Napoleon found the stability he had craved. He had a steady job, he bought a house, and started a family. Eventually he was briefly elected to the state legislature, followed by an appointment as postmaster. Yet despite his success, he always felt inferior because of his disability. 'My physical condition

9   Todd Depastino, *Citizen Hobo: How a Century of Homelessness Shaped America* (Chicago: University of Chicago Press, 2003), p. 4; *The Soldier's Friend* (New York), June 1866; Perkins, *The Memoirs of N.B. Perkins*, pp. 25–36.
10   Donald C. Pfanz, *Richard S. Ewell: A Soldier's Life* (Chapel Hill, NC: University of North Carolina Press, 1998), p. 265; Perkins, *The Memoirs of N.B. Perkins*, p. 31.

has always been a great handicap in making my way in life,' he wrote. 'No one except those who have lost a leg as near the body as I have can realize what it means and no one except my wife knows the suffering I have endured.' Perkins' voice was just one among thousands of voices of disabled Civil War veterans who struggled to demonstrate that they were still men.[11]

11   Perkins, *The Memoirs of N.B. Perkins*, p. 36.

The First Amputee

James Edward Hanger (1843–1919) enlisted in the Confederate
Churchville Cavalry in 1861. His 'Record of Services' was written for
his daughter in March 1914, and is excerpted with the permission of
the Hanger Clinic. His wounding was recorded by Ambrose Bierce in
'On a Mountain.' 'I cannot look back upon those days in the hospital
without a shudder,' Hanger later said. 'No one can know what such
a loss means unless he has suffered a similar catastrophe. In the
twinkling of an eye, life's fondest hopes seemed dead. I was the prey
of despair. What could the world hold for a maimed, crippled man!'
After returning home, Hanger requested a room exclusively for his
own use. Unbeknown to his family, he secretly devised an artificial
limb for himself made from whittled barrel staves and willow with a
hinged knee and foot. He patented this limb in 1871 for his company,
J.E. Hanger, Inc., of Richmond Virginia, whose headquarters moved
to Washington, DC, in 1888. By the time of Hanger's death his
company had several branches in the United States as well as in
London and Paris. The company has worked closely with the War
and Navy Departments and the Veterans Administration. To this
day the Hanger Orthopedic Group continues to play a leading role
in prosthetics.

   See 'The J.E. Hanger Story' at http://www.hanger.com/history/
Pages/The-J.E.-Hanger-Story.aspx.

Two columns were approaching Philippi [West Virginia] from the west on two
roads; the third column was to circumvent the town and cut off our retreat, in
which they almost succeeded. The heavy roads and a little incident which I'll
relate kept them from bagging our entire command. A pistol shot at or about
4.30 was to be the signal for the battery to commence firing. This battery had
been placed on a high hill just west of the town about 2 o'clock that morning.

   As the col[umn] on the Clarksburg road passed old Mrs. Humphreys'
home about 2 miles from Philippi just about daybreak, she started one of her

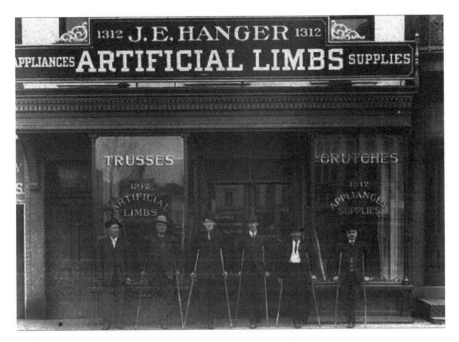

Figure 9: The J.E. Hanger shop front

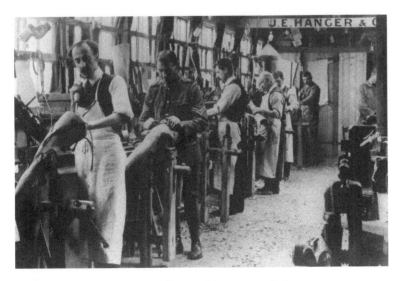

Figure 10: The J.E. Hanger workshop

boys to notify our command. Her boy was captured by some stragglers and she fired a gun at them. The commander of the battery took this for the signal and commenced firing about 4.20. He told me this. This firing was the first notice we had that the enemy was near us. The col[umn] that was to cut off our retreat was delayed some 30 or 40 minutes on account of heavy roads, which gave our forces time to get away.

The first two shots were canister and directed at the Cavalry Camps; the third shot was a six pound solid shot aimed at a stable in which the Churchville Cavalry company had slept. This shot struck the ground, richochetted, entering the stable and struck me. I remained in the stable till they came in there looking for plunder, about 4 hours after I was wounded. My limb was amputated by DR. Robinson, 16th Ohio Vol. I was taken to a private house in Philippi, was well taken care of. I remained there 2 weeks and was then taken out to Mr. Tom Hite's 3 miles from Philippi. I was exchanged at Norfolk about the last of August, 1861. My limb was the first amputation of the war.

Testimonial Letter

During the 1860s prosthetic limbs became big business. Promotional pamphlets included testimonials from their wearers, like the following from Lieutenant George Warner (27th Reg. Massachusetts Volunteers), which appeared in *Reporter of the New Patent Artificial Leg, Published by D. DeForest Douglas, Inventor and Manufacturer* (Springfield, MA: J.F. Tannatt, 1863).

Dear Sir, March 14th, 1862 and Sept. 22d, 1862, are two eventful periods in the history of my life. At the memorable battle of Newbern, N.C., while in command of a company, my right leg was carried away by a grape shot. As soon as was practicable I sought your skill and aid, and on the 22d of September commenced wearing your unequalled Patent Artificial Leg.

Previous to this time, I was besought and besieged by leg makers in New York, to procure their substitutes, even offering them at a less price than yours.

In examining the various kinds of Legs, I could readily distinguish the *superiority* of yours, by the difference of construction from others. I could easily see it is the most *durable, reliable,* and *substantial,* and the most natural in its movements, of any Leg invented.

That you have been eminently successful in its application in my case, I will say, I walk anywhere, and that without a cane. I have been hunting all day at a time, loading and firing my gun with the greatest facility and precision. I have walked as far through the woods, tramping up hill and down, over logs and through the brush, as my comrades.

I find the operation under all circumstances, natural, and *perfectly reliable.* The fitting and bearing are perfectly easy. Its mode of adjustment is *superior* to anything I have ever seen. It is finely ventilated, keeping the stump cool and healthy. My friends are surprised to see with what ease and freedom of motion I walk. They are unable to detect the artificial from the natural foot.

I would most earnestly and cheerfully advise my comrades who have lost their legs in defence of our country, to avail themselves of your *unequalled*

Artificial Leg, knowing that by so doing they will realize their anticipations, and be treated in the most successful manner.

To show you the facility with which I am using my limb, and my confidence in its reliability, I will add that today I leave for Newbern, to rejoin my Regiment, and resume active service in the field.

The Salem Leg (brochure)

From *The Salem Leg: Under the Patronage of the United States Government for the Use of the Army and the Navy* (Salem, MA: Office of the Salem Leg Company, 1864).

This original, simple, and elegant leg, is now manufactured by the Salem Leg Company, which has established its Office and Manufactory at. No. 26 Lynde St. Salem, Mass. The legs are manufactured under the immediate superintendence of the Inventor and Patentee – Prof. Geo. B. Jewett of Salem – who does not claim to have made an improvement on any particular limb or limbs now before the public, but to have originated a method of constructing artificial legs, which is essentially different from all other methods, and in many respects not only really, but obviously superior. This superiority is not found in any single peculiarity, but in many features of the invention, as will appear under the head of 'Advantages.' The Inventor has been using these limbs for nearly three years; and the opinion frequently expressed to him by surgeons and others, of the best judges, who have witnessed its action in conferring an easy, natural, and graceful step, fully justifies him in challenging a comparison of results, in these particulars, with any wearer of an artificial limb made in this country, or in Europe.

The Inventor of this leg having learned, from painful experience, that *wood* – the material commonly used for sockets – was entirely unsuitable tor his case determined to select such materials, not merely tor the socket but for every part of the leg, as were best adapted to secure the ends in view, namely, *comfort, strength, durability, convenience, economy and elegance.* Accordingly the *Salem Leg is NOT a wooden leg.* It has two sockets, one of yielding material, which is shaped over a cast of the stump, and another of sheet metal, which serves as a light, firm, yet slightly elastic case for the soft socket. The exterior, or metallic socket, is mounted on steel supporters, which, uniting at a suitable distance below the stump, are connected with a screw proceeding from the joint. The joints are of steel, and are so constructed as to secure *steadiness, smoothness* and *silence* of action. The action at the joints is limited by shoulders and cushions, all cords being dispensed with. The shaping up of the leg is done with hair and other suitable materials; and the covering is of flesh-colored leather, so attached that it can be removed or replaced with little inconvenience or expense. The whole leg is so put together that it may be *taken apart, readjusted* and *reconstructed*, with the utmost facility.

The brochure lists no fewer than 25 advantages.

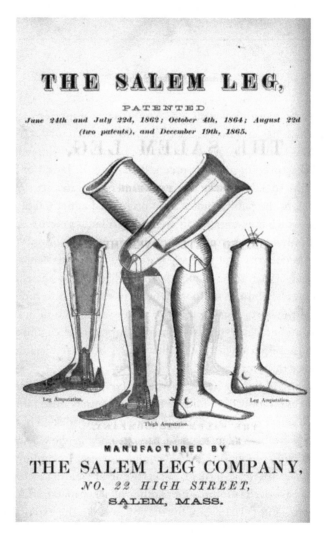

Figure 11: The Salem Leg

Testimony of Wearers

The following 'cases' are taken from 'Testimony of Wearers' in *The Salem Leg*. See also Guy R. Hasegawa, *Mending Broken Soldiers: The Union and Confederate Programs to Supply Artificial Limbs* (Carbondale, IL: Southern Illinois University Press, 2013).

Case B.

Thigh amputation. 'Stands at work for eight hours a day, without trouble or inconvenience. Frequently walks a mile or two afterwards in the evening. Can walk four or five miles without pain or fatigue. Does not use a cane, feels almost as secure from falling or tripping as with the natural limb.'

Case C.

Leg amputation. Short and crooked stump. After two or three months' experience in the use of the artificial leg, could walk twelve miles a day.

Case D.

Leg amputation. Tall and heavy person. Short stump. During the first summer after receiving the leg, *mowed* for six or seven days.

Case E.

Leg amputation. Heavy person. Short stump. Had worn wooden sockets several years, which were abandoned from the day of receiving the Salem Leg. Speaks of the relief as 'thoroughly enjoyable.' Describes the suffering caused by the *wooden socket* and the *band of leather* around the thigh as 'agony' and 'torture.'

The Human Wheel

Oliver Wendell Holmes (1809–1894) was a physician and poet, famous for his 'Breakfast-Table' sketches. He was an ardent supporter of the Union cause and his son Oliver Wendell Holmes, Jr. saw extensive military service in the war, which is recorded in Mark De Wolfe Howe, ed., *Touched with Fire: Civil War Letters and Diary of Oliver Wendell Holmes, Jr. 1861–1864* (Cambridge, MA: Harvard University Press, 1947). The elder Holmes became personally involved in the war when he received the following telegram about his son: 'Capt H wounded shot through the neck thought not mortal at Keedysville.' He later recorded his reactions: '*Through* the neck – no bullet left in wound. Windpipe, food-pipe, carotid, jugular, half a dozen smaller, but still formidable, vessels, a great braid of nerves, each as big as a lamp-wick, spinal cord – ought to kill at once, if at all. *Thought not* mortal, or *not thought* mortal – which was it?' The only answer was for him to find his son, as recorded in 'My Hunt for "The Captain,"' *Atlantic Monthly* 10 (December 1862), pp. 738–63.

Holmes Sr.'s essay 'The Human Wheel, Its Spokes and Felloes,' excerpted below, combines an examination of the 'mechanism of walking' with a celebration of American inventors – particularly Plumer and Palmer – whose products were increasingly in demand as a result of injuries in the war. He attacks the peg leg as inadequate and the crutch as 'at best an instrument of torture.' Holmes politicizes the new design for an artificial leg as a sign of US cultural independence and an example of the nation's capacity to combine utility with aesthetic appeal.

J.C. Plumer designed boots and shoes based on the anatomical principles of the foot, which were supplied to the army. B. Frank Palmer similarly designed artificial arms and legs, which were also supplied to the army. The Palmer Leg was patented in 1846, Palmer founding the American Artificial Limb Company. For a promotional pamphlet on the latter, see *The Palmer Arm and Leg, Adapted for the U.S. Army and Navy by the Surgeon-General, U.S.A.* (1865), at https://archive.org/details/101462403.nlm.nih.gov.

For further reading see David D. Yuan, 'Disfigurement and Reconstruction in Oliver Wendell Holmes's "The Human Wheel, Its Spokes and Felloes,"' in David T. Mitchell and Sharon L. Snyder, eds, *The Body and Physical Difference: Discourses of Disability* (Ann Arbor, MI: University of Michigan Press, 1997), pp. 70–88. Veteran Samuel Decker designed his own prosthetic arm in 1865, which was recorded through photographs taken in the Army Medical Museum. The museum described his arm as 'an apparatus hitherto unrivaled for its ingenuity and utility.' See Plate 20.

'The Human Wheel, Its Spokes and Felloes' was first published in *The Atlantic Monthly* 63 (May 1863), pp. 567–80, and was collected in Oliver Wendell Holmes, *Soundings from the Atlantic* (Boston: Ticknor and Fields, 1864).

The starting-point of this paper was a desire to call attention to certain remarkable AMERICAN INVENTIONS, especially to one class of mechanical contrivances, which, at the present time, assumes a vast importance and interests great multitudes. The limbs of our friends and countrymen are a part of the melancholy harvest which War is sweeping down [...] The admirable contrivances of an American inventor, prized as they were in ordinary times, have risen into the character of a great national blessing since the necessity for them has become so widely felt. While the weapons that have gone from Mr. Colt's armories have been carrying death to friend and foe, the beneficent and ingenious inventions of MR. PALMER have been repairing the losses inflicted by the implements of war.

[...]

Man is a *wheel*, with two spokes, his legs, and two fragments of a tire, his feet. He *rolls* successively on each of these fragments from the heel to the toe. If he had spokes enough, he would go round and round as the boys do when they 'make a wheel' with the four limbs for its spokes. But having only two available for ordinary locomotion, each of these has to be taken up as soon as it is used, and carried forward to be used again, and so alternatively with the pair. The peculiarity of biped-walking is, that the centre of gravity is shifted from one leg to the other, and the one not employed can shorten itself so as to swing forward, passing by that which supports the body.

[*Holmes gives a physiological account of walking and praises recent developments in footwear and the design of artificial limbs. – ed.*]

American taste was offended, outraged by the odious 'peg' which Old-World soldier or beggar was proud to show. We owe the well-shaped, intelligent, docile limb, the half-reasoning willow of Mr. Palmer to the same sense of beauty and fitness which moulded the soft outlines of the Indian Girl and the White Captive in the studio of his name-sake at Albany [*allusions to the American sculptor Erastus Dow Palmer – ed.*]. As we wean ourselves from the Old World, and become more and more nationalized in our great struggle for existence as a free people, we shall carry the aptness for beautiful forms more and more into common life, which demands first what is necessary and then what is pleasing.

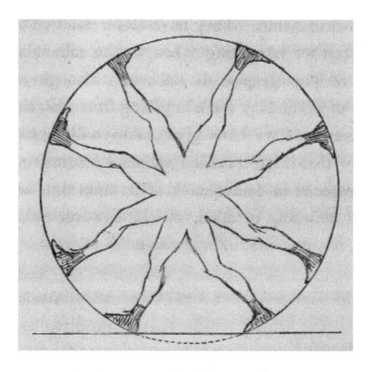

Figure 12: 'The Human Wheel'

The Case of George Dedlow

Silas Weir Mitchell (1829–1914), was a Philadelphia physician, invited in 1863 to co-direct the Turner's Lane Hospital for nervous diseases in Philadelphia by the Surgeon General of the US Army. He later recorded that 'new modes of treatment were devised, and gymnastic classes instituted, under the care of intelligent sergeants of the invalid corps; electricity was constantly employed, and hypodermic medication – at that time somewhat novel – was habitually resorted to, and its effects carefully studied'; in *Injuries of Nerves and their Consequences* (Philadelphia: J.B. Lippincott, 1872), pp. 10–11.

Mitchell became a pioneer of the study of neurology and 'causalgia,' identifying the 'phantom limb' sensation experienced by amputees and dramatized in the story above. The 'stump hospital' was the popular name for the South Street Hospital in Philadelphia, so called because of their large number of amputations.

'The Case of George Dedlow' first appeared anonymously in *The Atlantic Monthly* of July 1866, collected in *The Autobiography of a Quack and Other Stories* (New York: The Century Company, 1900), with the following introduction:

'The Case of George Dedlow' was not written with any intention that it should appear in print. I lent the manuscript to the Rev. Dr. Furness and forgot it. This gentleman sent it to the Rev. Edward Everett Hale. He, presuming, I fancy, that every one desired to appear in the Atlantic, offered it to that journal. To my surprise, soon afterwards I received a proof and a check. The story was inserted as a leading article without my name. It was at once accepted by many as the description of a real case. Money was collected in several places to assist the unfortunate man, and benevolent persons went to the 'Stump Hospital,' in Philadelphia, to see the sufferer and to offer him aid. The spiritual incident at the end of the story was received with joy by the spiritualists as a valuable proof of the truth of their beliefs.

The following notes of my own case have been declined on various pretexts by every medical journal to which I have offered them. There was, perhaps, some reason in this, because many of the medical facts which they record are not altogether new, and because the psychical deductions to which they have led me are not in themselves of medical interest. I ought to add, that a good deal of what is here related is not of any scientific value whatsoever; but as one or two people on whose judgment I rely have advised me to print my narrative with all the personal details, rather than in the dry shape in which, as a psychological statement, I shall publish it elsewhere, I have yielded to their views. I suspect, however, that the very character of my record will, in the eyes of some of my readers, tend to lessen the value of the metaphysical discoveries which it sets forth.

* * *

I am the son of a physician, still in large practice, in the village of Abington, Scofield County, Indiana. Expecting to act as his future partner, I studied medicine in his office, and in 1859 and 1860 attended lectures at the Jefferson Medical College in Philadelphia. My second course should have been in the following year, but the outbreak of the Rebellion so crippled my father's means that I was forced to abandon my intention. The demand for army surgeons at this time became very great; and although not a graduate, I found no difficulty in getting the place of Assistant-Surgeon to the Tenth Indiana Volunteers. In the subsequent Western campaigns this organization suffered so severely, that, before the term of its service was over, it was merged in the Twenty-First Indiana Volunteers; and I, as an extra surgeon, ranked by the medical officers of the latter regiment, was transferred to the Fifteenth Indiana Cavalry. Like many physicians, I had contracted a strong taste for army life, and, disliking cavalry service, sought and obtained the position of First-Lieutenant in the Seventy-Ninth Indiana Volunteers – an infantry regiment of excellent character.

On the day after I assumed command of my company, which had no captain, we were sent to garrison a part of a line of block-houses stretching along the Cumberland River below Nashville, then although occupied by a portion of the command of General Rosecrans.

The life we led while on this duty was tedious, and at the same time dangerous in the extreme. Food was scarce and bad, the water horrible, and we had no cavalry to forage for us. If, as infantry, we attempted to levy supplies upon the scattered farms around us, the population seemed suddenly to double, and in the shape of guerrillas 'potted' us industriously from behind distant trees, rocks, or hasty earthworks. Under these various and unpleasant influences, combined with a fair infusion of malaria, our men rapidly lost health and spirits. Unfortunately, no proper medical supplies had been forwarded with our small force (two companies), and, as the fall advanced, the want of quinine and stimulants became a serious annoyance. Moreover, our rations were running low; we had been three weeks without a new supply; and our commanding officer, Major Terrill, began to be uneasy as to the safety of his men. About this time it was supposed that a train with rations would be due from the post twenty miles to the north of us; yet it was quite possible that it would bring us food, but no medicines, which were what we most needed. The command was too small to detach any part of it, and the major therefore resolved to send an officer alone to the post above us, where the rest of the Seventy-ninth lay, and whence they could easily forward quinine and stimulants by the train, if it had not left, or, if it had, by a small cavalry escort.

It so happened, to my cost, as it turned out, that I was the only officer fit to make the journey, and I was accordingly ordered to proceed to Blockhouse No. 3 and make the required arrangements. I started alone just after dusk the next night, and during the darkness succeeded in getting within three miles of my destination. At this time I found that I had lost my way, and, although aware of the danger of my act, was forced to turn aside and ask at a log cabin for directions. The house contained a dried-up old woman and four white-headed, half-naked children. The woman was either stone-deaf or pretended to be so; but, at all events, she gave me no satisfaction, and I remounted and rode away. On coming to the end of a lane, into which I had turned to seek the cabin, I found to my surprise that the bars had been put up during my brief parley. They were too high to leap, and I therefore dismounted to pull them down. As I touched the top rail, I heard a rifle, and at the same instant felt a blow on both arms, which fell helpless. I staggered to my horse and tried to mount; but, as I could use neither arm, the effort was vain, and I therefore stood still, awaiting my fate. I am only conscious that I saw about me several graybacks, for I must have fallen fainting almost immediately.

When I awoke, I was lying in the cabin near by, upon a pile of rubbish. Ten or twelve guerrillas were gathered about the fire, apparently drawing lots for my watch, boots, hat, etc. I now made an effort to find out how far I was hurt. I discovered that I could use the left forearm and hand pretty well, and with this hand I felt the right limb all over until I touched the wound. The ball had passed from left to right through the left biceps, and directly through the right arm just below the shoulder, emerging behind. The right hand and forearm were cold and perfectly insensible. I pinched them as well as I could, to test the amount of sensation remaining; but the hand might as well have been that of a dead man. I began to understand that the nerves had been wounded, and that the part was utterly powerless. By this time my friends had pretty well divided the spoils, and, rising together, went out. The old woman then came to me and said, 'Reckon you'd best git up. Theyuns is agoin' to take you away.' To this I only answered, 'Water, water.' I had a grim sense of amusement on finding that the old woman was not deaf, for she went out, and presently came back with a gourdful, which I eagerly drank. An hour later the Graybacks returned, and, finding that I was too weak to walk, carried me out, and laid me on the bottom of a common cart, with which they set off on a trot. The jolting was horrible, but within an hour I began to have in my dead right hand a strange burning, which was rather a relief to me. It increased as the sun rose and the day grew warm, until I felt as if the hand was caught and pinched in a red-hot vice. Then in my agony I begged my guard for water to wet it with, but for some reason they desired silence, and at every noise threatened me with a revolver. At length the pain became absolutely unendurable, and I grew what it is the fashion to call demoralized. I screamed, cried, and yelled in my torture, until, as I suppose, my captors became alarmed, and, stopping, gave me a handkerchief – my own, I fancy – and a canteen of water, with which I wetted the hand, to my unspeakable relief.

It is unnecessary to detail the events by which, finally, I found myself in one of the Rebel hospitals near Atlanta. Here, for the first time, my wounds were properly cleansed and dressed by a Dr. Oliver Wilson, who treated me throughout with great kindness. I told him I had been a doctor; which, perhaps, may have been in part the cause of the unusual tenderness with which I was managed. The left arm was now quite easy; although, as will be seen, it never entirely healed. The right arm was worse than ever – the humerus broken, the nerves wounded, and the hand only alive to pain. I use this phrase because it is connected in my mind with a visit from a local visitor – I am not sure he was a preacher – who used to go daily through the wards, and talk to us, or write our letters. One morning he stopped at my bed, when this little talk occurred.

'How are you, Lieutenant?'

'O,' said I, 'as usual. All right, but this hand, which is dead except to pain.'

'Ah,' said he, 'such and thus will the wicked be – such will you be if you die in your sins: you will go where only pain can be felt. For all eternity, all of you will be as that hand – knowing pain only.'

I suppose I was very weak, but somehow I felt a sudden and chilling horror of possible universal pain, and suddenly fainted. When I awoke, the hand was worse, if that could be. It was red, shining, aching, burning, and, as it seemed to me, perpetually rasped with hot files. When the doctor came, I begged for morphia. He said gravely: 'We have none. You know you don't allow it to pass the lines.'

I turned to the wall, and wetted the hand again, my sole relief. In about an hour, Dr. Wilson came back with two aids, and explained to me that the bone was so broken as to make it hopeless to save it, and that, besides, amputation offered some chance of arresting the pain. I had thought of this before, but the anguish I felt – I cannot say endured – was so awful, that I made no more of losing the limb than of parting with a tooth on account of toothache. Accordingly, brief preparations were made, which I watched with a sort of eagerness such as must forever be inexplicable to any one who has not passed six weeks of torture like that which I had suffered.

I had but one pang before the operation. As I arranged myself on the left side, so as to make it convenient for the operator to use the knife, I asked: 'Who is to give me the ether?' 'We have none,' said the person questioned. I set my teeth, and said no more.

I need not describe the operation. The pain felt was severe; but it was insignificant as compared to that of any other minute of the past six weeks. The limb was removed very near to the shoulder-joint. As the second incision was made, I felt a strange lightning of pain play through the limb, defining every minutest fibril of nerve. This was followed by instant, unspeakable relief, and before the flaps were brought together I was sound asleep. I have only a recollection that I said, pointing to the arm which lay on the floor: 'There is the pain, and here am I. How queer!' Then I slept – slept the sleep of the just, or, better, of the painless. From this time forward, I was free from neuralgia; but at a subsequent period I saw a number of cases similar to mine in a hospital in Philadelphia.

It is no part of my plan to detail my weary months of monotonous prison life in the South. In the early part of August, 1863, I was exchanged, and, after the usual thirty days' furlough, returned to my regiment a captain.

On the 19th of September, 1863, occurred the battle of Chickamauga, in which my regiment took a conspicuous part. The close of our own share in this contest is, as it were, burnt into my memory with every least detail. It was about six P.M., when we found ourselves in line, under cover of a long, thin row of scrubby trees, beyond which lay a gentle slope, from which, again, rose a hill rather more abrupt, and crowned with an earthwork. We received orders to cross this space, and take the fort in front, while a brigade on our right was to make a like movement on its flank.

Just before we emerged into the open ground, we noticed what, I think, was common in many fights – that the enemy had begun to bowl round-shot at us, probably from failure of shell. We passed across the valley in good order, although the men fell rapidly all along the line. As we climbed the hill, our pace slackened, and the fire grew heavier. At this moment a battery opened on our left – the shots crossing our heads obliquely. It is this moment which is so printed on my recollection. I can see now, as if through a window, the gray smoke, lit with red flashes – the long, wavering line – the sky blue above – the trodden furrows, blotted with blue blouses. Then it was as if the window closed, and I knew and saw no more. No other scene in my life is thus scarred, if I may say so, into my memory. I have a fancy that the horrible shock which suddenly fell upon me must have had something to do with thus intensifying the momentary image then before my eyes.

When I awakened, I was lying under a tree somewhere at the rear. The ground was covered with wounded, and the doctors were busy at an operating-table, improvised from two barrels and a plank. At length two of them who were examining the wounded about me came up to where I lay. A hospital steward raised my head, and poured down some brandy and water, while another cut loose my pantaloons. The doctors exchanged looks, and walked away. I asked the steward where I was hit.

'Both thighs,' said he; 'the Doc's won't do nothing.'

'No use?' said I.

'Not much,' said he.

'Not much means none at all,' I answered.

When he had gone, I set myself to thinking about a good many things which I had better have thought of before, but which in no way concern the history of my case. A half-hour went by. I had no pain, and did not get weaker. At last, I cannot explain why, I began to look about me. At first, things appeared a little hazy; but I remember one which thrilled me a little, even then.

A tall, blond-bearded major walked up to a doctor near me, saying, 'When you've a little leisure, just take a look at my side.'

'Do it now,' said the doctor.

The officer exposed his left hip. 'Ball went in here, and out here.'

The doctor looked up at him with a curious air – half pity, half amazement. 'If you've got any message, you'd best send it by me.'

'Why, you don't say it's serious?' was the reply.

'Serious! Why, you're shot through the stomach. You won't live over the day.'

Then the man did what struck me as a very odd thing. 'Anybody got a pipe?' Some one gave him a pipe. He filled it deliberately, struck a light with a flint, and sat down against a tree near to me. Presently the doctor came over to him, and asked what he could do for him.

'Send me a drink of Bourbon.'

'Anything else?'

'No.'

As the doctor left him, he called him back. 'It's a little rough, Doc, isn't it?'

No more passed, and I saw this man no longer, for another set of doctors were handling my legs, for the first time causing pain. A moment after, a steward put a towel over my mouth, and I smelt the familiar odor of chloroform, which I was glad enough to breathe. In a moment the trees began to move around from left to right – then faster and faster; then a universal grayness came before me, and I recall nothing further until I awoke to consciousness in a hospital-tent. I got hold of my own identity in a moment or two, and was suddenly aware of a sharp cramp in my left leg. I tried to get at it to rub it with my single arm, but, finding myself too weak, hailed an attendant. 'Just rub my left calf,' said I, 'if you please.'

'Calf?' said he, 'you ain't none, pardner. It's took off.'

'I know better,' said I. 'I have pain in both legs.'

'Wall, I never!' said he. 'You ain't got nary leg.'

As I did not believe him, he threw off the covers, and, to my horror, showed me that I had suffered amputation of both thighs, very high up.

'That will do,' said I, faintly.

A month later, to the amazement of every one, I was so well as to be moved from the crowded hospital at Chattanooga to Nashville, where I filled one of the ten thousand beds of that vast metropolis of hospitals. Of the sufferings which then began I shall presently speak. It will be best just now to detail the final misfortune which here fell upon me. Hospital No. 2, in which I lay, was inconveniently crowded with severely wounded officers. After my third week, an epidemic of hospital gangrene broke out in my ward. In three days it attacked twenty persons. Then an inspector came out, and we were transferred at once to the open air, and placed in tents. Strangely enough, the wound in my remaining arm, which still suppurated, was seized with gangrene. The usual remedy, bromine, was used locally, but the main artery opened, was tied, bled again and again, and at last, as a final resort, the remaining arm was amputated at the shoulder-joint. Against all chances I recovered, to find myself a useless torso, more like some strange larval creature than anything of human shape. Of my anguish and horror of myself I dare not speak. I have dictated these pages, not to shock my readers, but to possess them with facts in regard to the relation of the mind to the body; and I hasten, therefore, to such portions of my case as best illustrate these views.

In January, 1864, I was forwarded to Philadelphia, in order to enter what was then known as the Stump Hospital, South Street. This favor was obtained through the influence of my father's friend, the late Governor Anderson, who has always manifested an interest in my case, for which I am deeply grateful. It was thought, at the time, that Mr. Palmer, the leg-maker, might be able to adapt some form of arm to my left shoulder, as on that side there remained five inches of the arm bone, which I could move to a moderate extent. The hope proved illusory, as the stump was always too tender to bear any pressure. The hospital referred to was in charge of several surgeons while I was an inmate, and was at all times a clean and pleasant home. It was filled with men who had lost one arm or leg, or one of each, as happened now and then. I saw one man who had lost both legs, and one who had parted with both arms; but none, like myself, stripped of every limb. There were collected in this place hundreds of these cases, which gave to it, with reason enough, the not very pleasing title of Stump-Hospital.

I spent here three and a half months, before my transfer to the United States Army Hospital for nervous diseases. Every morning I was carried out in an arm-chair, and placed in the library, where some one was always ready to write or read for me, or to fill my pipe. The doctors lent me medical books; the ladies brought me luxuries, and fed me; and, save that I was helpless to a degree which was humiliating, I was as comfortable as kindness could make me.

I amused myself, at this time, by noting in my mind all that I could learn from other limbless folk, and from myself, as to the peculiar feelings which were noticed in regard to lost members. I found that the great mass of men who had undergone amputations, for many months felt the usual consciousness that they still had the lost limb. It itched or pained, or was cramped, but never felt hot or cold. If they had painful sensations referred to it, the conviction of its existence continued unaltered for long periods; but where no pain was felt in it, then, by degrees, the sense of having that limb faded away entirely. I think we may to some extent explain this. The knowledge we possess of any part is made up of the numberless impressions from without which affect its sensitive surfaces, and which are transmitted through its nerves to the spinal nerve-cells, and through them, again, to the brain. We are thus kept endlessly informed as to the existence of parts, because the impressions which reach the brain are, by a law of our being, referred by us to the part from which they came. Now, when the part is cut off, the nerve-trunks which led to it and from it, remaining capable of being impressed by irritations, are made to convey to the brain from the stump impressions which are as usual referred by the brain to the lost parts, to which these nerve-threads belonged. In other words, the nerve is like a bell-wire. You may pull it at any part of its course, and thus ring the bell as well as if you pulled at the end of the wire; but, in any case, the intelligent servant will refer the pull to the front door, and obey it accordingly. The impressions made on the cut ends of the nerve, or on its sides, are due often to the changes in the stump during healing, and consequently cease as it heals, so that finally, in a very healthy stump, no such impressions arise; the brain ceases to correspond with the lost leg, and, as les absents ont toujours tort, it is no longer remembered or recognized. But in some cases, such as mine proved at last to my sorrow, the ends of the nerves undergo a curious alteration, and get to be enlarged and altered. This change, as I have seen in my practice of medicine, passes up the nerves towards the centres, and occasions a more or less constant irritation of the nerve-fibres, producing neuralgia, which is usually referred to that part of the lost limb to which the affected nerve belongs. This pain keeps the brain ever mindful of the missing part, and, imperfectly at least, preserves to the man a consciousness of possessing that which he has not.

Where the pains come and go, as they do in certain cases, the subjective sensations thus occasioned are very curious, since in such cases the man loses and gains, and loses and regains, the consciousness of the presence of lost parts, so that he will tell you, 'Now I feel my thumb – now I feel my little finger.' I should also add, that nearly every person who has lost an arm above the elbow feels as though the lost member were bent at the elbow, and at times is vividly impressed with the notion that his fingers are strongly flexed.

Another set of cases present a peculiarity which I am at a loss to account for. Where the leg, for instance, has been lost, they feel as if the foot was present, but as though the leg were shortened. If the thigh has been taken off, there seems to them to be a foot at the knee; if the arm, a hand seems to be at the elbow, or attached to the stump itself.

As I have said, I was next sent to the United States Army Hospital for Injuries and Diseases of the Nervous System. Before leaving Nashville, I had begun to suffer the most acute pain in my left hand, especially the little finger; and so perfect was the idea which was thus kept up of the real presence of these missing parts, that I found it hard at times to believe them absent. Often, at night, I would try with one lost hand to grope for the other. As, however, I had no pain in the right arm, the sense of the existence of that limb gradually disappeared, as did that of my legs also.

Everything was done for my neuralgia which the doctors could think of; and at length, at my suggestion, I was removed to the above-named hospital. It was a pleasant, suburban, old-fashioned country-seat, its gardens surrounded by a circle of wooden, one-story wards, shaded by fine trees. There were some three hundred cases of epilepsy, paralysis, St. Vitus's dance, and wounds of nerves. On one side of me lay a poor fellow, a Dane, who had the same burning neuralgia with which I once suffered, and which I now learned was only too common. This man had become hysterical from pain. He carried a sponge in his pocket, and a bottle of water in one hand, with which he constantly wetted the burning hand. Every sound increased his torture, and he even poured water into his boots to keep himself from feeling too sensibly the rough friction of his soles when walking. Like him, I was greatly eased by having small doses of morphia injected under the skin of my shoulder, with a hollow needle, fitted to a syringe.

As I improved under the morphia treatment, I began to be disturbed by the horrible variety of suffering about me. One man walked sideways; there was one who could not smell; another was dumb from an explosion. In fact, every one had his own abnormal peculiarity. Near me was a strange case of palsy of the muscles called rhomboids, whose office it is to hold down the shoulder-blades flat on the back during the motions of the arms, which, in themselves, were strong enough. When, however, he lifted these members, the shoulder-blades stood out from the back like wings, and got him the sobriquet of the 'Angel.' In my ward were also the cases of fits, which very much annoyed me, as upon any great change in the weather it was common to have a dozen convulsions in view at once. Dr. Neek, one of our physicians, told me that on one occasion a hundred and fifty fits took place within thirty-six hours. On my complaining of these sights, whence I alone could not fly, I was placed in the paralytic and wound ward, which I found much more pleasant.

A month of skilful treatment eased me entirely of my aches, and I then began to experience certain curious feelings, upon which, having nothing to do and nothing to do anything with, I reflected a good deal. It was a good while before I could correctly explain to my own satisfaction the phenomena which at this time I was called upon to observe. By the various operations already described I had lost about four fifths of my weight. As a consequence of this I ate much less than usual, and could scarcely have consumed the ration of a soldier. I slept also but little; for, as sleep is the repose of the brain, made necessary by the waste of its tissues during thought and voluntary movement, and as this latter did not exist in my case, I needed only that rest which was necessary to repair such exhaustion of the nerve-centers as was induced by thinking and the automatic movements of the viscera.

I observed at this time also that my heart, in place of beating, as it once did, seventy-eight in the minute, pulsated only forty-five times in this interval – a fact to be easily explained by the perfect quiescence to which I was reduced, and the consequent absence of that healthy and constant stimulus to the muscles of the heart which exercise occasions.

Notwithstanding these drawbacks, my physical health was good, which, I confess, surprised me, for this among other reasons: It is said that a burn of two thirds of the surface destroys life, because then all the excretory matters which this portion of the glands of the skin evolved are thrown upon the blood, and poison the man, just as happens in an animal whose skin the physiologist has varnished, so as in this way to destroy its function. Yet here was I, having lost at least a third of my skin, and apparently none the worse for it.

Still more remarkable, however, were the psychical changes which I now began to perceive. I found to my horror that at times I was less conscious of myself, of my own existence, than used to be the case. This sensation was so novel that at first it quite bewildered me. I felt like asking some one constantly if I were really George Dedlow or not; but, well aware how absurd I should seem after such a question, I refrained from speaking of my case, and strove more keenly to analyze my feelings. At times the conviction of my want of being myself was overwhelming and most painful. It was, as well as I can describe it, a deficiency in the egoistic sentiment of individuality. About one half of the sensitive surface of my skin was gone, and thus much of relation to the outer world destroyed. As a consequence, a large part of the receptive central organs must be out of employ, and, like other idle things, degenerating rapidly. Moreover, all the great central ganglia, which give rise to movements in the limbs, were also eternally at rest. Thus one half of me was absent or functionally dead. This set me to thinking how much a man might lose and yet live. If I were unhappy enough to survive, I might part with my spleen at least, as many a dog has done, and grown fat afterwards. The other organs with which we breathe and circulate the blood would be essential; so also would the liver; but at least half of the intestines might be dispensed with, and of course all of the limbs. And as to the nervous system, the only parts really necessary to life are a few small ganglia. Were the rest absent or inactive, we should have a man reduced, as it were, to the lowest terms, and leading an almost vegetative existence. Would such a being, I asked myself, possess the sense of individuality in its usual completeness, even if his organs of sensation remained, and he were capable of consciousness? Of course, without them, he could not have it any more than a dahlia or a tulip. But with them – how then? I concluded that it would be at a minimum, and that, if utter loss of relation to the outer world were capable of destroying a man's consciousness of himself, the destruction of half of his sensitive surfaces might well occasion, in a less degree, a like result, and so diminish his sense of individual existence.

I thus reached the conclusion that a man is not his brain, or any one part of it, but all of his economy, and that to lose any part must lessen this sense of his own existence. I found but one person who properly appreciated this great truth. She was a New England lady, from Hartford – an agent, I think, for some commission, perhaps the Sanitary. After I had told her my views and feelings she said: 'Yes, I comprehend. The fractional entities of vitality are embraced in the oneness of the unitary Ego. Life,' she added, 'is the garnered condensation of objective impressions; and as the objective is the remote father of the subjective, so must individuality, which is but focused subjectivity, suffer and fade when the sensation lenses, by which the rays of impression are condensed, become destroyed.' I am not quite clear that I fully understood her, but I think she appreciated my ideas, and I felt grateful for her kindly interest.

The strange want I have spoken of now haunted and perplexed me so constantly that I became moody and wretched. While in this state, a man from a neighboring ward fell one morning into conversation with the chaplain, within ear-shot of my chair. Some of their words arrested my attention, and I turned my head to see and listen. The speaker, who wore a sergeant's chevron and carried one arm in a sling was a tall, loosely made person, with a pale face, light eyes of a washed-out blue tint, and very sparse yellow whiskers. His mouth was weak, both lips being almost alike, so that the organ might have been turned upside down without affecting its expression. His forehead, however, was high and thinly covered with sandy hair. I should have said, as a phrenologist, will feeble; emotional, but not passionate; likely to be an enthusiast or a weakly bigot.

I caught enough of what passed to make me call to the sergeant when the chaplain left him.

'Good morning,' said he. 'How do you get on?'

'Not at all,' I replied. 'Where were you hit?'

'Oh, at Chancellorsville. I was shot in the shoulder. I have what the doctors call paralysis of the median nerve, but I guess Dr. Neek and the lightnin' battery will fix it. When my time's out I'll go back to Kearsarge and try on the school-teaching again. I've done my share.'

'Well,' said I, 'you're better off than I.'

'Yes,' he answered, 'in more ways than one. I belong to the New Church. It's a great comfort for a plain man like me, when he's weary and sick, to be able to turn away from earthly things and hold converse daily with the great and good who have left this here world. We have a circle in Coates street. If it wa'n't for the consoling I get there, I'd of wished myself dead many a time. I ain't got kith or kin on earth; but this matters little, when one can just talk to them daily and know that they are in the spheres above us.'

'It must be a great comfort,' I replied, 'if only one could believe it.'

'Believe!' he repeated. 'How can you help it? Do you suppose anything dies?'

'No,' I said. 'The soul does not, I am sure; and as to matter, it merely changes form.'

'But why, then,' said he, 'should not the dead soul talk to the living? In space, no doubt, exist all forms of matter, merely in finer, more ethereal being. You can't suppose a naked soul moving about without a bodily garment – no creed teaches that; and if its new clothing be of like substance to ours, only of ethereal fineness – a more delicate recrystallization about the eternal spiritual nucleus – must it not then possess powers as much more delicate and refined as is the new material in which it is reclad?'

'Not very clear,' I answered; 'but, after all, the thing should be susceptible of some form of proof to our present senses.'

'And so it is,' said he. 'Come to-morrow with me, and you shall see and hear for yourself.'

'I will,' said I, 'if the doctor will lend me the ambulance.'

It was so arranged, as the surgeon in charge was kind enough, as usual, to oblige me with the loan of his wagon, and two orderlies to lift my useless trunk.

On the day following I found myself, with my new comrade, in a house in Coates street, where a 'circle' was in the daily habit of meeting. So soon as I had been comfortably deposited in an arm-chair, beside a large pine table, the rest of those assembled seated themselves, and for some time preserved an unbroken silence. During this pause I scrutinized the persons present. Next to me, on my right, sat a flabby man, with ill-marked, baggy features and injected eyes. He was, as I learned afterwards, an eclectic doctor, who had tried his hand at medicine and several of its quackish variations, finally settling down on eclecticism, which I believe professes to be to scientific medicine what vegetarianism is to common-sense, every-day dietetics. Next to him sat a female-authoress, I think, of two somewhat feeble novels, and much pleasanter to look at than her books. She was, I thought, a good deal excited at the prospect of spiritual revelations. Her neighbor was a pallid, care-worn young woman, with very red lips, and large brown eyes of great beauty. She was, as I learned afterwards, a magnetic patient of the doctor, and had deserted her husband, a master mechanic, to follow this new light. The others were, like myself, strangers brought hither by mere curiosity. One of them was a lady in deep black, closely veiled. Beyond her, and opposite to me, sat the sergeant, and next to him the medium, a man named Brink. He wore a good deal of jewelry, and had large black side-whiskers – a shrewd-visaged, large-nosed, full-lipped man, formed by nature to appreciate the pleasant things of sensual existence.

Before I had ended my survey, he turned to the lady in black, and asked if she wished to see any one in the spirit-world.

She said, 'Yes,' rather feebly.

'Is the spirit present?' he asked. Upon which two knocks were heard in affirmation. 'Ah!' said the medium, 'the name is – it is the name of a child. It is a male child. It is –'

'Alfred!' she cried. 'Great Heaven! My child! My boy!'

On this the medium arose, and became strangely convulsed. 'I see,' he said, 'I see – a fair-haired boy. I see blue eyes – I see above you, beyond you –' at the same time pointing fixedly over her head.

She turned with a wild start. 'Where – whereabouts?'

'A blue-eyed boy,' he continued, 'over your head. He cries – he says, "Mama, mama!"'

The effect of this on the woman was unpleasant. She stared about her for a moment, and exclaiming, 'I come – I am coming, Alfy!' fell in hysterics on the floor.

Two or three persons raised her, and aided her into an adjoining room; but the rest remained at the table, as though well accustomed to like scenes. After this several of the strangers were called upon to write the names of the dead with whom they wished to communicate. The names were spelled out by the agency of affirmative knocks when the correct letters were touched by the applicant, who was furnished with an alphabet-card upon which he tapped the letters in turn, the medium, meanwhile, scanning his face very keenly. With some, the names were readily made out. With one, a stolid personage of disbelieving type, every attempt failed, until at last the spirits signified by knocks that he was a disturbing agency, and that while he remained all our efforts would fail. Upon this some of the company proposed that he should leave; of which invitation he took advantage, with a skeptical sneer at the whole performance.

As he left us, the sergeant leaned over and whispered to the medium, who next addressed himself to me. 'Sister Euphemia,' he said, indicating the lady with large eyes, 'will act as your medium. I am unable to do more. These things exhaust my nervous system.'

'Sister Euphemia,' said the doctor, 'will aid us. Think, if you please, sir, of a spirit, and she will endeavor to summon it to our circle.'

Upon this a wild idea came into my head. I answered: 'I am thinking as you directed me to do.'

The medium sat with her arms folded, looking steadily at the center of the table. For a few moments there was silence. Then a series of irregular knocks began. 'Are you present?' said the medium.

The affirmative raps were twice given.

'I should think,' said the doctor, 'that there were two spirits present.'

His words sent a thrill through my heart.

'Are there two?' he questioned.

A double rap.

'Yes, two,' said the medium. 'Will it please the spirits to make us conscious of their names in this world?'

A single knock. 'No.'

'Will it please them to say how they are called in the world of spirits?'

Again came the irregular raps – 3, 4, 8, 6; then a pause, and 3, 4, 8, 7.

'I think,' said the authoress, 'they must be numbers. Will the spirits,' she said, 'be good enough to aid us? Shall we use the alphabet?'

'Yes,' was rapped very quickly.

'Are these numbers?'

'Yes,' again.

'I will write them,' she added, and, doing so, took up the card and tapped the letters. The spelling was pretty rapid, and ran thus as she tapped, in turn, first the letters, and last the numbers she had already set down:

'UNITED STATES ARMY MEDICAL MUSEUM, Nos. 3486, 3487.'

The medium looked up with a puzzled expression.

'Good gracious!' said I, 'they are MY LEGS – MY LEGS!'

What followed, I ask no one to believe except those who, like myself, have communed with the things of another sphere. Suddenly I felt a strange return of my self-consciousness. I was reindividualized, so to speak. A strange wonder filled me, and, to the amazement of every one, I arose, and, staggering a little, walked across the room on limbs invisible to them or me. It was no wonder I staggered, for, as I briefly reflected, my legs had been nine months in the strongest alcohol. At this instant all my new friends crowded around me in astonishment. Presently, however, I felt myself sinking slowly. My legs were going, and in a moment I was resting feebly on my two stumps upon the floor. It was too much. All that was left of me fainted and rolled over senseless.

I have little to add. I am now at home in the West, surrounded by every form of kindness and every possible comfort; but alas! I have so little surety of being myself that I doubt my own honesty in drawing my pension, and feel absolved from gratitude to those who are kind to a being who is uncertain of being enough himself to be conscientiously responsible. It is needless to add that I am not a happy fraction of a man, and that I am eager for the day when I shall rejoin the lost members of my corporeal family in another and a happier world.

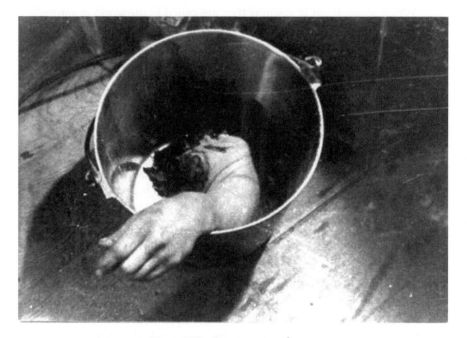

Figure 13: An amputated arm

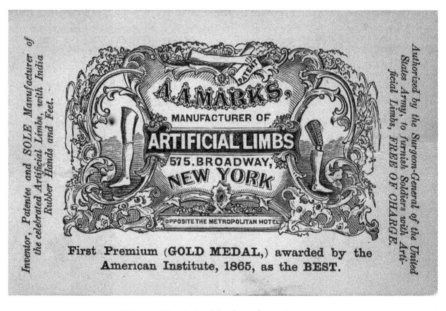

Figure 14: A.A. Marks advertisement

Phantom Limbs

The following is from Silas Weir Mitchell's 'Phantom Limbs,' *Lippincott's Magazine of Popular Literature and Science* 8 (1871), pp. 563–69. Mitchell estimated that the war had produced at least 15,000 amputees, now known to be a gross under-estimate.

Mitchell extended his studies into everyday life with *Wear and Tear or, Hints for the Overworked* (1871), developing a rest cure which was taken by Charlotte Perkins Gilman (dramatized in her 1892 story 'The Yellow Wallpaper'), Edith Wharton, and later by Virginia Woolf. In his 1884 novel, *In War Time*, Mitchell describes the Filbert Street Hospital in Philadelphia. For commentary on his career, see Nancy Cervetti, *S. Weir Mitchell, 1829–1914: Philadelphia's Literary Physician* (University Park, PA: Pennsylvania University Press, 2012).

Many persons feel the lost limb as existing the moment they awaken from the merciful stupor of the ether given to destroy the torments of the knife; others come slowly to this consciousness in days or weeks, and when the wound has healed; but, as a rule, the more sound and serviceable the stump, especially if an artificial limb be worn, the more likely is the man to feel faintly the presence of the shorn member. Sometimes a blow on the stump will reawaken such consciousness, or, as happened in one case, a reamputation higher up the limb will summon it anew into seeming existence.

In many, the limb may be recalled to the man by irritating the nerves in its stump. Every doctor knows that when any part of a nerve is excited by the excited by a pinch, a tap or by electricity – which is an altogether harmless means – the pain, if it be a nerve of feeling, is felt as if it were really caused in the part to which the nerve finally passes.

[...]

On one occasion the shoulder was thus electrized three inches above the point where the arm had been cut off. For two years the man had ceased to be conscious of the limb. As the current passed, although ignorant of its possible effects, he started up, crying aloud, 'Oh, the hand, the hand!' and trying to seize it with the living grasp of the sound fingers. No resurrection of the dead, no answer of a summoned spirit, could have been more startling. As the current was broken the lost part faded again, only to be recalled by the same means. This man had ceased to feel his limb. With others it is a presence never absent save in sleep.

[...]

Perhaps the oddest of all phenomena which may follow amputation is the gradual shortening which the patient imagines to be undergone by the phantom limb. In a certain proportion of instances of removal of a member above the knee or elbow, the lost arm or leg begins to lose length very early, and by a gradual process the hand at length seems to be set at the elbow or the foot at the knee. All sense of the intervening parts is lost, and in rare cases the hand appears to be actually imbedded in the stump. A patient describing this condition insisted that the stump felt less distinctly present than the hand, which, for him, appeared to lie in the stump, save that the finger-ends projected beyond it. At this point the hand remained, and has moved no further.

[...]

In full health we receive in the brain, when we move a part, impression as to the force exerted, the position gained, and the like, which are messages from the part moved, and which at once become of value in regulating, directing or checking the movement. The nerves which carry such information to the conscious brain when electrized in the stump convey at once to the head sensations which, seeming to come from the muscles of the lost limb, create in the brain the illusion of their having moved.

IN THE FIELD OF BATTLE

Diary:

October 29, 1862

Henry Tisdale (1837–1922) enlisted in the 35th regiment of the Massachusetts Volunteer Infantry, saw extensive action, and was captured by the Rebels 1864–65. His diary is transcribed by family members. Taken from Mark F. Farrell, ed., *The Civil War Diary and Letters of Sergeant Henry W. Tisdale* (2001), at http://civilwardiary.net © 2001. Excerpted with permission.

Some six weeks have passed away since writing. They have been eventful ones to me, full of God's providential goodness and mercy. A good deal of the time I have been unable to write and the remaining time I have been indisposed to it. At near 4 PM September 14th our brigade was ordered to the front, a rough march of some 4 miles brought us to the scene of conflict, climbing steep hills, some almost mountains crossing rough fields through corn fields and some of the way at double quick. On our way meeting many wounded being carried to the rear and as we neared the battleground here and there a dead body was to be seen. At little after 5 PM were upon the ground where the booming of artillery the screaming of shot and shell and rattling of musketry told us we were mid the stern realities of actual battle. The sight of the wounded sent a kind of chill over me but in the main feelings of curiosity and wonder at the scene about me took hold of my mind. Were drawn up in the line of battle in a cornfield and then advanced through a sort of wooden field to a thick wood where we met the rebels or a few scattering ones for their main body was on the retreat. In entering the wood came upon a large number of rebel dead lying in a ravine, presenting a sad and sickening sight. They were making an advance upon our lines, but when crossing the ravine, were met by a volley from the 17th Michigan which so thinned their ranks that on that part of their line they made a precipitate retreat. Just after we entered the wood was wounded by a rifle ball passing through my left leg just opposite the thighbone. As the ball struck me it gave me a shock which led me to feel at first that the bone must have been struck and shattered and for a moment did not dare to move for fear it was so. Found on moving that the bone was not injured and that I had only a flesh wound, which relieved my mind and thankfulness to God that I was not maimed or dangerously hurt came. I think that the shot must have been fired by some straggling rebel or sharpshooter in a tree, as we had not yet got up to within reach of the rebel lines. Found myself in a few moments growing weak and tying my towel above the wound to stop its bleeding tried to make for the rear where the surgeons were. As I was limping off a wounded rebel who was sitting against a tree called me and asked me if I did not have something to eat. Exhibiting a loaf and going to him I opened my knife to cut off a slice when he placed his hands before his face exclaiming 'Don't kill me' and begging me to put up the knife and not to hurt him. Assuring him I had no intention of hurting him I spoke with him a little. Found he had a family in Georgia, that he was badly wounded and was anxious to have me remain with him and help him off. But found I was growing weaker from loss of blood and that the surging to and fro the troops about us made it a dangerous place so limping and crawling was obliged to leave him and move for the rear. Soon came across some men detailed to look out for the wounded who placed me in a blanket and took me to the rear to the surgeon. The place where the wounded were brought was near a cottage, near which had been the battle-ground of the forenoon. Was fortunate enough to be placed upon a straw bed in the garden just outside the house and had my wound promptly dressed. The cottage had a memento of the fight in the shape of a hole through its roof made by a cannon ball. The fighting continued till late in the evening, our regiment losing but a few wounded among them our colonel lost his left arm and George E. Whiting of our company one of his feet. He bore the amputation manfully. The house and outbuildings and the ground adjoining them were filled and covered with wounded rebel and union mingled, all being cared for as best they could be, many moaning piteously throughout the night or until death put an end to their sufferings. Friend Sabin R. Baker of our company took care of us of the regiment doing what he could and adding much to our comfort amid the confusion and suffering existing about. On the afternoon of Tuesday Sept. 16th a train of ambulances came and all of us able to be moved were taken to Middletown and placed in the churches vacant dwelling etc. in town. Endeavored to get into the same building with Whiting but in vain. Was saddened to hear while at Frederick, MD of his death, from dysentery and weakness from his wound. Remained at Middletown until the next afternoon; the citizens generously supplying us with food and other needs; when we were moved to Frederick, and were placed in the Lutheran Church, which was turned into a hospital. A rough board floor was laid over the tops of the pews. Folding iron bedsteads with mattresses, clean white sheets, pillows, blankets, and clean underclothing, hospital dressing gowns, slippers, etc. were furnished us freely. The citizens came in twice a day with a host of luxuries, cordials, etc. for our comfort. The church finely finished off within, well ventilated and our situation as pleasant and comfortable as could be made. A few rebel wounded were in the building. Some of the citizens showed them special attention bringing them articles of food, etc. and giving none to the others. The surgeons put a stop to this however by telling them that they must distribute to all alike or they would not be allowed to visit the hospital at all, this was much to our satisfaction. Remained in Frederick until Sept. 30th, getting on slowly, having my wound dressed twice a day. A liberal supply of reading material and other comforts furnished by the citizens – when able to go about on crutches was sent off for Philadelphia. Had a rough ride thither, were placed in box freight cars with but a thin layer of straw upon the floor to lie upon. Owing to delays were 27 hours on the trip. Were kindly cared for on arrival at Philadelphia at the Citizen's Volunteer Hospital and from thence was transferred to a regular government hospital at the corner of 5th and Burtonwood Streets. Here I found every appliance that humanity could suggest for our comfort. Was placed in the 4th story of the building. Wound continued to heal nicely giving me but little pain and in about a fortnight was able to hobble about the room and dress myself and by the 20th of October to walk out doors. Found many sad cases of wounds and sickness in the hospital, many from shattered limbs had been lying for many months slowly recovering and waiting to be able to be sent home./

The Battle of Shiloh:

Aftermath

The following is taken from Colonel Willis De Hass, 'The Battle of Shiloh,' *Annals of the War Written by Leading Participants North and South*, ed. Alexander Kelly McClure (Philadelphia: Times Publishing Co., 1979). The pieces in this collection were originally published in the *Philadelphia Weekly Times*. In the introduction, the editor declares that the *Annals* will 'furnish the most valuable contributions to the future historian which have yet given to the world.'

Gradually the firing ceased. The Sabbath closed upon a scene which had no parallel on the Western Continent. The sun went down in a red halo, as if the very heavens blushed and prepared to weep at the enormity of man's violence. Night fell upon and spread its funereal pall over a field of blood where death held unrestrained carnival! Soon after dark the rain descended in torrents, and all through the dreary hours of that dismal night it rained unceasingly. The groans of the dying, and the solemn thunder of the gunboats came swelling at intervals high above the peltings of the pitiless storm.

[...]

The dead were buried on the spot; the wounded removed to camp; the rebel camp destroyed, with a large amount of property, and this was the last of the fighting at Shiloh. The losses sustained by both armies exceeded the frightful number of twenty-five thousand men. Four years after the battle, a writer, visiting Shiloh and Corinth, gave a hideous picture of the condition of things. He stated that twelve thousand Confederate soldiers lay unburied on the two fields! After the battle of Shiloh, General Grant ordered the dead of both armies to be buried. The inhumation, however, consisted of little more than a thin covering of earth, which the heavy rains have long since washed off, and the remains of brave men, who periled all for their country's sake, he exposed to the elements. This fact is disgraceful to the government and the people, and should be remedied with the least possible delay. Instead of squandering means over idle parades, it should be our duty and pleasure to give the bleaching bones of our gallant dead the rites of decent burial. Regarding this as fitting opportunity, it is respectfully and earnestly suggested that Congress adopt some measure for the preservation of the remains at Shiloh – that a cemetery be established, and graves properly marked; also, that the church at Shiloh be rebuilt as a national memorial!

The Battle of Ellyson's Mills

The following is from Spencer Glasgow Welch, *A Confederate Surgeon's Letters to His Wife* (New York and Washington: Neal Pub. Co., 1911). Welch was a surgeon in the 13th South Carolina Volunteers. The letters were edited by the surgeon's daughter, President of the Daughters of the Confederacy for the State of South Carolina.

June 3, 1862. On Sunday I was sent to Richmond to look after our sick and did not return until late yesterday afternoon. While there I had an opportunity to observe the shocking results of a battle, but, instead of increasing my horror of a battlefield, it made me more anxious than ever to be in a conflict and share its honours. To me every wounded man seemed covered with glory.

Our casualties were certainly very great, for every house which could be had was being filled with the wounded. Even the depots were being filled with them and they came pouring into the hospitals by wagon loads. Nearly all were covered with mud, as they had fought in a swamp most of the time and lay out all night after being wounded. Many of them were but slightly wounded, many others severely, large numbers mortally, and some would die on the road from the battlefield. In every direction the slightly wounded were seen with their arms in slings, their heads tied up, or limping about. One man appeared as if he had been entirely immersed in blood, yet he could walk. Those in the hospitals had received severe flesh wounds or had bones broken, or some vital part penetrated. They did not seem to suffer much and but few ever groaned, but they will suffer when the reaction takes place. I saw one little fellow whose thigh was broken. He was a mere child, but was very cheerful.

Aftermath of Battle,

Cedar Mountain, Virginia

David Hunter Strother (1816–1888) was an American author and magazine illustrator, published under the pen-name of 'Porte Crayon,' i.e. 'Pencil Carrier,' probably a homage to Washington Irving's pen-name of Geoffrey Crayon. From 1866 to 1868 he published a series of eleven sketches in *Harper's Monthly* under the title 'Personal Recollections of the War.' He joined the Union army as a topographer, rising in the ranks to brigadier-general.

In his opening sketch (June 1866) he records how the war initially struck him as the 'rage of adverse dogmatisms,' but then came to realize the large issues of freedom at stake. Of his 'Personal Recollections' he states: 'It will be seen that in writing these individual experiences it is not proposed to emulate the dignity and comprehensiveness of History, but to give closer and more detailed views of characters and events, a series of photographic pictures hastily caught during the action of the changing drama.' His attention to visual specifics comes out clearly in the excerpts above, which serve as a reminder that not all the fatalities in the war were human.

The following excerpt is from Strother's 'Personal Recollections of the War: Eighth Paper,' *Harper's New Monthly Magazine* 35 (June–November 1867), pp. 273–95.

I was sent forward with an order to hasten Buford's advance. Having delivered my message I took the opportunity of riding over the late battlefield. On the spot where the evening's advance fell upon the Staff on Saturday night, afterward occupied by one of their batteries, I saw fourteen dead bodies of horses, swelled and corrupting, in close contiguity. There were also four dead bodies of artillerists, supposed to be a captain, a lieutenant, and two privates. There were altogether twenty-seven horses lying in the vicinity, and the field and road were stained with blood and covered with scattered hats, equipments, broken wheels, and vehicles. The wood behind was terribly shattered by our artillery fire, not among the tree-tops, as is usually the case; but all our missiles seem to have struck near the ground, with an accuracy fatal to any body of infantry which may have occupied the wood as a support for the artillery. The effect of the fire was further indicated by the quantities of blood-stained rags, clothes, and equipments that lay in the woods [...] Passing through this wood I crossed a brook, and observed the open ground beyond strewed with broken belts, cartridge-boxes, knapsacks, bayonet-scabbards, blood-stained blankets, overcoats, hats, and shoes. The shoes had apparently been left by the rebels who exchanged with our dead and wounded. There were a few graves here and there of our men and officers buried where they fell.

[Exploring farther the following day]

Reviewing the ground lately described we rode over the spaces where the bloodiest contest had occurred, and beyond to the lines occupied by the enemy. The dead men were all buried; but the bodies of at least a hundred horses lay scattered over the field, and the stench was insupportable. The ground was rutted in every direction with the wheels of the artillery, and thickly strewed with *debris*. The graves and trenches we saw did not seem to indicate the large number of dead reported.

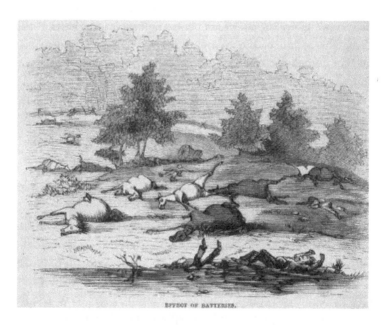

Figure 15: David Hunter Strother: 'The effect of batteries'

After the Battle of Winchester

The next excerpt is also by David Hunter Strother, taken from *A Virginia Yankee in the Civil War: The Diaries of David Hunter Strother*, edited with an introduction by Cecil D. Eby, Jr. © 1961 by the University of North Carolina Press. Used by permission of the publisher (www.uncpress.unc.edu). This edition presents Strother's original diaries and demonstrates the elaborate recasting process which went into his 'Personal Recollections.'

Last night I visited the courthouse [*in Winchester – ed.*] where a number of wounded of both armies lay. In the courtyard were two pieces of cannon, twelve-pounders, taken from the enemy. In the vestibule lay thirteen dead bodies of United States soldiers and the courtroom was filled to its capacity with wounded, all of a serious character. A Confederate captain, Yancey Jones, was lying there with both eyes scooped out and the bridge of his nose carried away by a bullet. He was sometimes delirious and roared about forming his company and charging. An Ohio volunteer lay on his back, the brains oozing from a shot in the head, uttering at breathing intervals a sharp stertorous cry. He had been lying thus for thirty-six hours. A few stifled groans were heard occasionally, but as a general thing the men were quiet. There was another storeroom opposite Taylor's Hotel where we saw a number of wounded, all Federalists.

This morning I visited the Union Hotel where I saw two rooms filled with wounded and seven dead. In the room where the dead bodies were, lay a Confederate soldier wounded in the head. He seemed also delirious and was rolling a piece of lint in his hands and rubbing the floor with it. He also pulled the bloody bandages from his head and the soldier nurse told us that he occasionally got up and ran about so violently that he was obliged to bring him out from among the other wounded. In the next room was a fairhaired man whose fixed eyes and stertorous breathing showed him to be in the agonies of death. Some here were lightly wounded in the limbs and one with a broken thigh showed me the wound and begged I would have it attended to. George

Washington of Jefferson County was upstairs said to be mortally wounded. At the door I met a lady [asking] for permission to visit him....

[...]

From the commencement of the attack on Saturday evening until Sunday evening the women of Winchester were insolently triumphant. They confidently expected to see the United States troops driven out and as the dead and wounded were brought in during the day, these Rebel dames and maids were on the streets and at the windows radiant with anticipated triumph, insulting the soldiers on duty in the town and the families of officers who were there visiting their husbands. As the evening closed, the scene changed. Ambulances came in carrying their own wounded by scores, and escorts with long trains of Rebel prisoners marched through the streets. The she-braggarts disappeared from the streets, doors were closed, and lights put out. Anon, veiled mourners besieged the doors of the hospitals and guard houses, begging permission to see a friend or husband among the wounded or prisoners. The cup of humiliation and sorrow is now at the lips of this insolent and inhuman race. Let them drain it to the dregs.

Christian Fleetwood,

The Negro as a Soldier

Christian Abraham Fleetwood (1840–1914) was a Baltimore-born African American who served in the US Coloured Infantry 1863–66, receiving the Medal of Honor for valour in battle. *The Negro as a Soldier* (Washington, DC: Howard University, 1895) was a pamphlet published for the Negro Congress of that year. Fleetwood was attempting to rectify a lack of attention to African American troops in the Civil War, partly through the memorializing image given below. Race theory was often incorporated in the assessment of soldiers. Roberts Bartholomew, for example, praised Americans for their toughness of muscular fibre, but believed that African Americans suffered from underdeveloped calves and flat feet, concluding that 'the Negro soldier is, unquestionably, less enduring than the white soldier' (Flint, ed., *Contributions to the Causation and Prevention*, p. 5).

[A]t the terrible mine explosion General B.F. Butler issued an order, a portion of which I quote, as follows:

'Of the colored soldiers of the third divisions of the 18th and 10th Corps and the officers who led them, the general commanding desires to make special mention. In the charge on the enemy's works by the colored division of the 18th Corps at New Market, better men were never better led, better officers never led, better men. A few more such gallant charges and to command colored troops will be the post of honor in the American armies. The colored soldiers, by coolness, steadiness, determined courage and dash, have silenced every cavil of the doubters of their soldierly capacity, and drawn tokens of admiration from their enemies, have brought their late masters even to the consideration of the question whether they will not employ as soldiers the hitherto despised race.'

Some ten or more years later, in Congress, in the midst of a speech advocating the giving of civil rights to the Negro, Gen. Butler said, referring to this incident [battle in 1864]:

'There, in a space not wider than the clerk's desk, and three hundred yards long, lay the dead bodies of 543 of my colored comrades, slain in the defense of their country, who had laid down their lives to uphold its flag and its honor, as a willing sacrifice. And as I rode along, guiding my horse this way and that, lest he should profane with his hoofs what seemed to me the sacred dead, and as I looked at their bronzed faces upturned in the shining sun, as if in mute appeal against the wrongs of the country for which they had given their lives, and whose flag had been to them a flag of stripes, in which no star of glory had ever shone for them – feeling I had wronged them in the past, and believing what was the future duty of my country to them – I swore to myself a solemn oath: "May my right hand forget its cunning, and my tongue cleave to the roof of my mouth, if ever I fail to defend the rights of the men who have given their blood for me and my country this day and for their race forever." And, God helping me, I will keep that oath.'

Thomas Wentworth Higginson,

Army Life in a Black Regiment

Thomas Wentworth Higginson (1823–1911) was a Unitarian minister and abolitionist. During the war he served as colonel in the 1st South Carolina Volunteers, the first regiment to be recruited from freed slaves. The Secretary of War stipulated that black regiments had to be commanded by white officers. Higginson was also one of the poet Emily Dickinson's correspondents. The following extract is taken from Higginson's *Army Life in a Black Regiment* (Boston: Fields, Osgood, 1870).

Introductory

I am under pretty heavy bonds to tell the truth, and only the truth; for those who look back to the newspaper correspondence of that period will see that this particular regiment lived for months in a glare of publicity, such as tests any regiment severely, and certainly prevents all subsequent romancing in its historian. As the scene of the only effort on the Atlantic coast to arm the negro, our camp attracted a continuous stream of visitors, military and civil. A battalion of black soldiers, a spectacle since so common, seemed then the most daring of innovations, and the whole demeanour of this particular regiment was watched with microscopic scrutiny by friends and foes. I felt sometimes as if we were a plant trying to take root, but constantly pulled up to see if we were growing. The slightest camp incidents sometimes came back to us, magnified and distorted, in letters of anxious inquiry from remote parts of the Union. It was no pleasant thing to live under such constant surveillance; but it guaranteed the honesty of any success, while fearfully multiplying the penalties had there been a failure. A single mutiny, such as has happened in the infancy of a hundred regiments, a single miniature Bull Run, a stampede of desertions, and it would have been all over with us; the party of distrust would have got the upper hand, and there might not have been, during the whole contest, another effort to arm the negro.

Camp Diary
December 29.

Our new surgeon has begun his work most efficiently: he and the chaplain have converted an old gin-house into a comfortable hospital, with ten nice beds and straw pallets. He is now, with a hearty professional faith, looking round for somebody to put into it. I am afraid the regiment will accommodate him; for, although he declares that these men do not sham sickness, as he expected, their catarrh is an unpleasant reality. They feel the dampness very much, and make such a coughing at dress-parade, that I have urged him to administer a dose of cough-mixture, all round, just before that pageant. Are the colored race *tough*? is my present anxiety; and it is odd that physical insufficiency, the only discouragement not thrown in our way by the newspapers, is the only discouragement which finds any place in our minds. They are used to sleeping indoors in winter, herded before fires, and so they feel the change. Still, the regiment is as healthy as the average, and experience will teach us something.

POST-WAR NARRATIVES

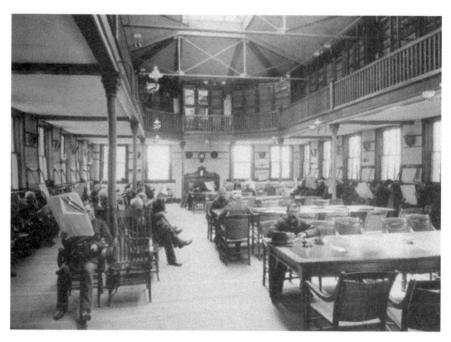

Figure 16: Library of the National Home for Veterans, Milwaukee

'What I Saw of Shiloh'

Later famous for his stories of the uncanny and for *The Devil's Dictionary*, originally titled *The Cynic's Wordbook* (1906), Ambrose Bierce (1842–1914?) enlisted in the Union army in 1861 and saw extensive action including the Battle of Shiloh in 1862. In 1864 he suffered a head wound in battle and was discharged from the army the following year. Virtually all his writing about the Civil War was retrospective. Bierce disappeared, probably in 1914, while serving in Mexico as an observer in Pancho Villa's army.

The following excerpt by Bierce was published in *The Wasp* (San Francisco), December 1881. The Battle of Shiloh took place in April 1862, appearing first to be a Confederate victory until the fortunes of war swung to the other side. For commentary, see Martin Buinicki and David Owens, 'De-Anthologizing Ambrose Bierce: A New look at "What I Saw of Shiloh,"' *War, Literature and the Arts* 23.i (2011), pp. 1–18. For further first-hand commentary on the Battle of Shiloh, see *MSHWR* Vol. 1, pp. 41–44.

In a few moments we had passed out of the singular oasis that had so marvelously escaped the desolation of battle, and now the evidences of the previous day's struggle were present in profusion. The ground was tolerably level here, the forest less dense, mostly clear of undergrowth, and occasionally opening out into small natural meadows. Here and there were small pools – mere discs of rainwater with a tinge of blood. Riven and torn with cannon-shot, the trunks of the trees protruded bunches of splinters like hands, the fingers above the wound interlacing with those below. Large branches had been lopped, and hung their green heads to the ground, or swung critically in their netting of vines, as in a hammock. Many had been cut clean off and their masses of foliage seriously impeded the progress of the troops. The bark of these trees, from the root upward to a height of ten or twenty feet, was so thickly pierced with bullets and grape that one could not have laid a hand on it without covering several punctures. None had escaped. How the human body survives a storm like this must be explained by the fact that it is exposed to it but a few moments at a time, whereas these grand old trees had had no one to take their places, from the rising to the going down of the sun. Angular bits of iron, concavo-convex, sticking in the sides of muddy depressions, showed where shells had exploded in their furrows. Knapsacks, canteens, haversacks distended with soaken and swollen biscuits, gaping to disgorge, blankets beaten into the soil by the rain, rifles with bent barrels or splintered stocks, waist-belts, hats and the omnipresent sardine-box – all the wretched debris of the battle still littered the spongy earth as far as one could see, in every direction. Dead horses were everywhere; a few disabled caissons, or limbers, reclining on one elbow, as it were; ammunition wagons standing disconsolate behind four or six sprawling mules. Men? There were men enough; all dead, apparently, except one, who lay near where I had halted my platoon to await the slower movement of the line – a Federal sergeant, variously hurt, who had been a fine giant in his time. He lay face upward, taking in his breath in convulsive, rattling snorts, and blowing it out in sputters of froth which crawled creamily down his cheeks, piling itself alongside his neck and ears. A bullet had clipped a groove in his skull, above the temple; from this the brain protruded in bosses, dropping off in flakes and strings. I had not previously known one could get on, even in this unsatisfactory fashion, with so little brain. One of my men, whom I knew for a womanish fellow, asked if he should put his bayonet through him. Inexpressibly shocked by the cold-blooded proposal, I told him I thought not; it was unusual, and too many were looking.

'The Coup de Grace'

The following text, also by Bierce, was published in the *San Francisco Examiner*, June 1889, and collected in *Tales of Soldiers and Civilians* (San Francisco: E.L.G. Steele, 1891), with the UK title *In the Midst of Life*.

The fighting had been hard and continuous; that was attested by all the senses. The very taste of battle was in the air. All was now over; it remained only to succor the wounded and bury the dead – to 'tidy up a bit,' as the humorist of a burial squad put it. A good deal of 'tidying up' was required. As far as one could see through the forests, among the splintered trees, lay wrecks of men and horses. Among them moved the stretcher-bearers, gathering and carrying away the few who showed signs of life. Most of the wounded had died of neglect while the right to minister to their wants was in dispute. It is an army regulation that the wounded must wait; the best way to care for them is to win the battle. It must be confessed that victory is a distinct advantage to a man requiring attention, but many do not live to avail themselves of it.

The dead were collected in groups of a dozen or a score and laid side by side in rows while the trenches were dug to receive them.

Some, found at too great a distance from these rallying points, were buried where they lay. There was little attempt at identification, though in most cases, the burial parties being detailed to glean the same ground which they had assisted to reap, the names of the victorious dead were known and listed. The enemy's fallen had to be content with counting. But of that they got enough: many of them were counted several times, and the total, as given afterward in the official report of the victorious commander, denoted rather a hope than a result.

At some little distance from the spot where one of the burial parties had established its 'bivouac of the dead,' a man in the uniform of a Federal officer stood leaning against a tree. From his feet upward to his neck his attitude was that of weariness reposing; but he turned his head uneasily from side to side; his mind was apparently not at rest. He was perhaps uncertain in which direction to go; he was not likely to remain long where he was, for already the level rays of the setting sun straggled redly through the open spaces of the wood and the weary soldiers were quitting their task for the day. He would hardly make a night of it alone there among scene the dead.

Nine men in ten whom you meet after a battle inquire the way to some fraction of the army – as if any one could know. Doubtless this officer was lost. After resting himself a moment he would presumably follow one of the retiring burial squads.

When all were gone he walked straight away into the forest toward the red west, its light staining his face like blood. The air of confidence with which he now strode along showed that he was on familiar ground; he had recovered his bearings. The dead on his right and on his left were unregarded as he passed. An occasional low moan from some sorely-stricken wretch whom the relief-parties had not reached, and who would have to pass a comfortless night beneath the stars with his thirst to keep him company, was equally unheeded. What, indeed, could the officer have done, being no surgeon and having no water?

At the head of a shallow ravine, a mere depression of the ground, lay a small group of bodies. He saw, and swerving suddenly from his course walked rapidly toward them. Scanning each one sharply as he passed, he stopped at last above one which lay at a slight remove from the others, near a clump of small trees. He looked at it narrowly. It seemed to stir. He stooped and laid his hand upon its face. It screamed.

The officer was Captain Downing Madwell, of a Massachusetts regiment of infantry, a daring and intelligent soldier, an honorable man.

In the regiment were two brothers named Halcrow – Caffal and Creede Halcrow. Caffal Halcrow was a sergeant in Captain Madwell's company, and these two men, the sergeant and the captain, were devoted friends. In so far as disparity of rank, difference in duties and considerations of military discipline would permit they were commonly together. They had, indeed, grown up together from childhood. A habit of the heart is not easily broken off. Caffal Halcrow had nothing military in his taste nor disposition, but the thought of separation from his friend was disagreeable; he enlisted in the company in which Madwell was second-lieutenant. Each had taken two steps upward in rank, but between the highest non-commissioned and the lowest commis-sioned officer the gulf is deep and wide and the old relation was maintained with difficulty and a difference.

Creede Halcrow, the brother of Caffal, was the major of the regiment – a cynical, saturnine man, between whom and Captain Madwell there was a natural antipathy which circumstances had nourished and strengthened to an active animosity. But for the restraining influence of their mutual relation to Caffal these two patriots would doubtless have endeavored to deprive their country of each other's services.

At the opening of the battle that morning the regiment was performing outpost duty a mile away from the main army. It was attacked and nearly surrounded in the forest, but stubbornly held its ground. During a lull in the fighting, Major Halcrow came to Captain Madwell. The two exchanged formal salutes, and the major said: 'Captain, the colonel directs that you push your company to the head of this ravine and hold your place there until recalled. I need hardly apprise you of the dangerous character of the movement, but if you wish, you can, I suppose, turn over the command to your first-lieutenant. I was not, however, directed to authorize the substitution; it is merely a suggestion of my own, unofficially made.'

To this deadly insult Captain Madwell coolly replied:

'Sir, I invite you to accompany the movement. A mounted officer would be a conspicuous mark, and I have long held the opinion that it would be better if you were dead.'

The art of repartee was cultivated in military circles as early as 1862.

A half-hour later Captain Madwell's company was driven from its position at the head of the ravine, with a loss of one-third its number. Among the fallen was Sergeant Halcrow. The regiment was soon afterward forced back to the main line, and at the close of the battle was miles away. The captain was now standing at the side of his subordinate and friend.

Sergeant Halcrow was mortally hurt. His clothing was deranged; it seemed to have been violently torn apart, exposing the abdomen. Some of the buttons of his jacket had been pulled off and lay on the ground beside him and fragments of his other garments were strewn about. His leather belt was parted and had apparently been dragged from beneath him as he lay. There had been no great effusion of blood. The only visible wound was a wide, ragged opening in the abdomen.

It was defiled with earth and dead leaves. Protruding from it was a loop of small intestine. In all his experience Captain Madwell had not seen a wound like this. He could neither conjecture how it was made nor explain the attendant circumstances – the strangely torn clothing, the parted belt, the besmirching of the white skin. He knelt and made a closer examination. When he rose to his feet, he turned his eyes in different directions as if looking for an enemy. Fifty yards away, on the crest of a low, thinly wooded hill, he saw several dark objects moving about among the fallen men – a herd of swine. One stood with its back to him, its shoulders sharply elevated. Its forefeet were upon a human body, its head was depressed and invisible. The bristly ridge of its chine showed black against the red west. Captain Madwell drew away his eyes and fixed them again upon the thing which had been his friend.

The man who had suffered these monstrous mutilations was alive. At intervals he moved his limbs; he moaned at every breath. He stared blankly into the face of his friend and if touched screamed. In his giant agony he had torn up the ground on which he lay; his clenched hands were full of leaves and twigs and earth. Articulate speech was beyond his power; it was impossible to know if he were sensible to anything but pain. The expression of his face was an appeal; his eyes were full of prayer. For what?

There was no misreading that look; the captain had too frequently seen it in eyes of those whose lips had still the power to formulate it by an entreaty for death. Consciously or unconsciously, this writhing fragment of humanity, this type and example of acute sensation, this handiwork of man and beast, this humble, unheroic Prometheus, was imploring everything, all, the whole non-ego, for the boon of oblivion. To the earth and the sky alike, to the trees, to the man, to whatever took form in sense or consciousness, this incarnate suffering addressed that silent plea.

For what, indeed? For that which we accord to even the meanest creature without sense to demand it, denying it only to the wretched of our own race: for the blessed release, the rite of uttermost compassion, the *coup de grâce*.

Captain Madwell spoke the name of his friend. He repeated it over and over without effect until emotion choked his utterance.

His tears plashed upon the livid face beneath his own and blinded himself. He saw nothing but a blurred and moving object, but the moans were more distinct than ever, interrupted at briefer intervals by sharper shrieks. He turned away, struck his hand upon his forehead, and strode from the spot. The swine, catching sight of him, threw up their crimson muzzles, regarding him suspiciously a second, and then with a gruff, concerted grunt, raced away out of sight. A horse, its foreleg splintered by a cannon-shot, lifted its head sidewise from the ground and neighed piteously. Madwell stepped forward, drew his revolver and shot the poor beast between the eyes, narrowly observing its death-struggle, which, contrary to his expectation, was violent and long; but at last it lay still. The tense muscles of its lips, which had uncovered the teeth in a horrible grin, relaxed; the sharp, clean-cut profile took on a look of profound peace and rest.

Along the distant, thinly wooded crest to westward the fringe of sunset fire had now nearly burned itself out. The light upon the trunks of the trees had faded to a tender gray; shadows were in their tops, like great dark birds aperch. Night was coming and there were miles of haunted forest between Captain Madwell and camp. Yet he stood there at the side of the dead animal, apparently lost to all sense of his surroundings. His eyes were bent upon the earth at his feet; his left hand hung loosely at his side, his right still held the pistol. Presently he lifted his face, turned it toward his dying friend and walked rapidly back to his side. He knelt upon one knee, cocked the weapon, placed the muzzle against the man's forehead, and turning away his eyes pulled the trigger. There was no report. He had used his last cartridge for the horse.

The sufferer moaned and his lips moved convulsively. The froth that ran from them had a tinge of blood.

Captain Madwell rose to his feet and drew his sword from the scabbard. He passed the fingers of his left hand along the edge from hilt to point. He held it out straight before him, as if to test his nerves. There was no visible tremor of the blade; the ray of bleak skylight that it reflected was steady and true. He stooped and with his left hand tore away the dying man's shirt, rose and placed the point of the sword just over the heart. This time he did not withdraw his eyes. Grasping the hilt with both hands, he thrust downward with all his strength and weight. The blade sank into the man's body – through his body into the earth; Captain Madwell came near falling forward upon his work. The dying man drew up his knees and at the same time threw his right arm across his breast and grasped the steel so tightly that the knuckles of the hand visibly whitened. By a violent but vain effort to withdraw the blade the wound was enlarged; a rill of blood escaped, running sinuously down into the deranged clothing. At that moment three men stepped silently forward from behind the clump of young trees which had concealed their approach. Two were hospital attendants and carried a stretcher.

The third was Major Creede Halcrow.

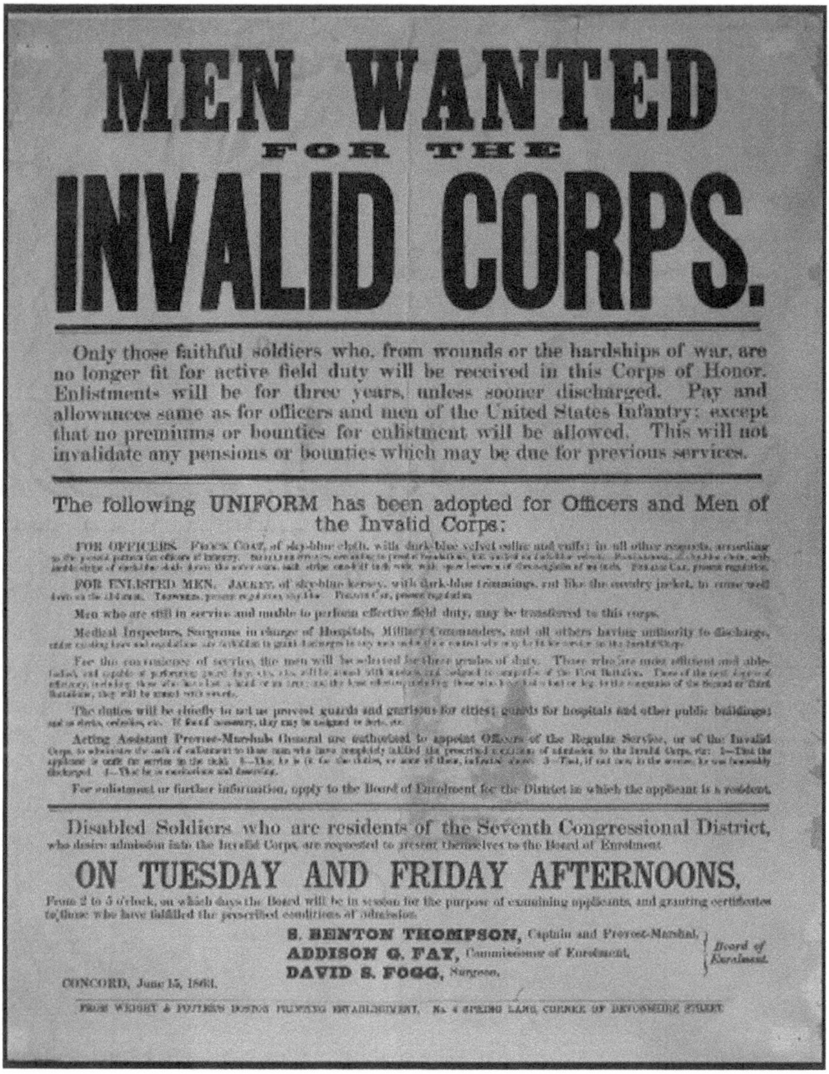

Figure 17: The Invalid Corps, 1863 poster

'A Resumed Identity'

Bierce's 'A Resumed Identity' was first published as 'The Man' in *The Cosmopolitan* (New York), September 1908, and collected in *Can Such Things Be?* (New York: Cassell, 1893). This is one of Bierce's tales that engages with the psychological damage of the war.

See also: Jim McWilliams, 'Ambrose Bierce's Civil War: One Man's Morbid Vision,' *Civil War Times* magazine, http://www. historynet.com/ambrose-bierces-civil-war-one-mans-morbid-vision. htm; Don Swaim, *Civil War Bierce*, http://donswaim.com/bierce-civilwar.html; Giorgio Mariani, 'Ambrose Bierce's Civil War Stories and the Critique of the Martial Spirit,' *Studies in American Fiction* 19.ii (Autumn 1991), pp. 221–28.

I – THE REVIEW AS A FORM OF WELCOME

One summer night a man stood on a low hill overlooking a wide expanse of forest and field. By the full moon hanging low in the west he knew what he might not have known otherwise: that it was near the hour of dawn. A light mist lay along the earth, partly veiling the lower features of the landscape, but above it the taller trees showed in well-defined masses against a clear sky. Two or three farmhouses were visible through the haze, but in none of them, naturally, was a light. Nowhere, indeed, was any sign or suggestion of life except the barking of a distant dog, which, repeated with mechanical iteration, served rather to accentuate than dispel the loneliness of the scene.

The man looked curiously about him on all sides, as one who among familiar surroundings is unable to determine his exact place and part in the scheme of things. It is so, perhaps, that we shall act when, risen from the dead, we await the call to judgment.

A hundred yards away was a straight road, showing white in the moonlight. Endeavoring to orient himself, as a surveyor or navigator might say, the man moved his eyes slowly along its visible length and at a distance of a quarter-mile to the south of his station saw, dim and gray in the haze, a group of horsemen riding to the north. Behind them were men afoot, marching in column, with dimly gleaming rifles aslant above their shoulders. They moved slowly and in silence. Another group of horsemen, another regiment of infantry, another and another – all in unceasing motion toward the man's point of view, past it, and beyond. A battery of artillery followed, the cannoneers riding with folded arms on limber and caisson. And still the interminable procession came out of the obscurity to south and passed into the obscurity to north, with never a sound of voice, nor hoof, nor wheel.

The man could not rightly understand: he thought himself deaf; said so, and heard his own voice, although it had an unfamiliar quality that almost alarmed him; it disappointed his ear's expectancy in the matter of *timbre* and resonance. But he was not deaf, and that for the moment sufficed.

[...]

II – WHEN YOU HAVE LOST YOUR LIFE CONSULT A PHYSICIAN

Dr. Stilling Malson, of Murfreesboro, having visited a patient six or seven miles away, on the Nashville road, had remained with him all night. At daybreak he set out for home on horseback, as was the custom of doctors of the time and region. He had passed into the neighborhood of Stone's River battlefield when a man approached him from the roadside and saluted in the military fashion, with a movement of the right hand to the hat-brim. But the hat was not a military hat, the man was not in uniform and had not a martial bearing. The doctor nodded civilly, half thinking that the stranger's uncommon greeting was perhaps in deference to the historic surroundings. As the stranger evidently desired speech with him he courteously reined in his horse and waited.

'Sir,' said the stranger, 'although a civilian, you are perhaps an enemy.'

'I am a physician,' was the non-committal reply.

'Thank you,' said the other. 'I am a lieutenant, of the staff of General Hazen.' He paused a moment and looked sharply at the person whom he was addressing, then added, 'Of the Federal army.'

The physician merely nodded.

'Kindly tell me,' continued the other, 'what has happened here. Where are the armies? Which has won the battle?'

The physician regarded his questioner curiously with half-shut eyes. After a professional scrutiny, prolonged to the limit of politeness, 'Pardon me,' he said; 'one asking information should be willing to impart it. Are you wounded?' he added, smiling.

'Not seriously – it seems.'

The man removed the unmilitary hat, put his hand to his head, passed it through his hair and, withdrawing it, attentively considered the palm.

'I was struck by a bullet and have been unconscious. It must have been a light, glancing blow: I find no blood and feel no pain. I will not trouble you for treatment, but will you kindly direct me to my command – to any part of the Federal army – if you know?'

Again the doctor did not immediately reply: he was recalling much that is recorded in the books of his profession – something about lost identity and the effect of familiar scenes in restoring it. At length he looked the man in the face, smiled, and said:

'Lieutenant, you are not wearing the uniform of your rank and service.'

At this the man glanced down at his civilian attire, lifted his eyes, and said with hesitation:

'That is true. I – I don't quite understand.'

Still regarding him sharply but not unsympathetically the man of science bluntly inquired:

'How old are you?'

'Twenty-three – if that has anything to do with it.'

'You don't look it; I should hardly have guessed you to be just that.'

The man was growing impatient. 'We need not discuss that,' he said; 'I want to know about the army. Not two hours ago I saw a column of troops moving northward on this road. You must have met them. Be good enough to tell me the color of their clothing, which I was unable to make out, and I'll trouble you no more.'

'You are quite sure that you saw them?'

'Sure? My God, sir, I could have counted them!'

'Why, really,' said the physician, with an amusing consciousness of his own resemblance to the loquacious barber of the Arabian Nights, 'this is very interesting. I met no troops.'

The man looked at him coldly, as if he had himself observed the likeness to the barber. 'It is plain,' he said, 'that you do not care to assist me. Sir, you may go to the devil!'

He turned and strode away, very much at random, across the dewy fields, his half-penitent tormentor quietly watching him from his point of vantage in the saddle till he disappeared beyond an array of trees.

III – THE DANGER OF LOOKING INTO A POOL OF WATER

After leaving the road the man slackened his pace, and now went forward, rather deviously, with a distinct feeling of fatigue. He could not account for this, though truly the interminable loquacity of that country doctor offered itself in explanation. Seating himself upon a rock, he laid one hand upon his knee, back upward, and casually looked at it. It was lean and withered. He lifted both hands to his face. It was seamed and furrowed; he could trace the lines with the tips of his fingers. How strange! – a mere bullet-stroke and a brief unconsciousness should not make one a physical wreck.

'I must have been a long time in hospital,' he said aloud. 'Why, what a fool I am! The battle was in December, and it is now summer!' He laughed. 'No wonder that fellow thought me an escaped lunatic. He was wrong: I am only an escaped patient.'

At a little distance a small plot of ground enclosed by a stone wall caught his attention. With no very definite intent he rose and went to it. In the center was a square, solid monument of hewn stone. It was brown with age, weather-worn at the angles, spotted with moss and lichen. Between the massive blocks were strips of grass the leverage of whose roots had pushed them apart. In answer to the challenge of this ambitious structure Time had laid his destroying hand upon it, and it would soon be 'one with Nineveh and Tyre.' In an inscription on one side his eye caught a familiar name. Shaking with excitement, he craned his body across the wall and read:

HAZEN'S BRIGADE
to
The Memory of Its Soldiers
who fell at
Stone River, Dec. 31, 1862.

The man fell back from the wall, faint and sick. Almost within an arm's length was a little depression in the earth; it had been filled by a recent rain – a pool of clear water. He crept to it to revive himself, lifted the upper part of his body on his trembling arms, thrust forward his head and saw the reflection of his face, as in a mirror. He uttered a terrible cry. His arms gave way; he fell, face downward, into the pool and yielded up the life that had spanned another life.

'Recollections of a Private'

Warren Lee Goss's 'Recollections of a Private' (1885) was published in *The Century Illustrated Monthly Magazine*, May to October 1885. *The Century* promoted the publication of Civil War memoirs in its 'Battles and Leaders of the Civil War' series, which ran from November 1884 to November 1887, massively increasing the magazine's subscription. Robert Underwood Johnson and Clarence Clough Buel edited *The Century*'s four-volume *Battles and Leaders of the Civil War* (New York: Century Company, 1887–88). Unsolicited memoirs of the war started appearing in 1885 under the title 'Memoranda on the Civil War,' brief pieces commenting on previous articles. An editorial comment on the series declared: 'when completed it will probably constitute a more authoritative and final statement of the events of the war as seen through the eyes of commanders and participants than has before been made on a single plan' (March 1885, p. 788).

Collected with other pieces as *Recollections of a Private. A Story of the Army of the Potomac* (New York: Thomas Y. Crowell, 1890). Goss's accounts are cumulative, combining reports from different eyewitnesses. In his preface to the 1890 collection he explained:

Herein I have endeavored to speak for my many comrades in the ranks. [...] The 'Army of the Potomac' was the people in arms. It mirrored the diversified opinions and occupations of a free and intelligent democracy. The force that called it together was the spirit that made a government of the people possible. Its ranks were largely filled with youth, who had no love for war, but who had left their pleasant homes, and the pursuits of peace, that the government they loved might not perish. To the large numbers of patriotic young men in the ranks is to be attributed much of its hopeful spirit. Thus it was that, though baffled by bloody and disheartening reverses, though it changed its commanders often, it never lost its discipline, its heroic spirit, or its confidence in final success. Its private soldiers were often as intelligent critics of military movements as were their superiors.

Goss published a number of works about young infantrymen, including *The Soldier's Story of His Captivity at Andersonville, Belle Isle, and Other Rebel Prisons* (1867).

Up the Peninsula with McClennan [from the Peninsula Campaign in Virginia, 1862]

In all the pictures of battles I had seen before I ever saw a battle, the officers were at the front on prancing steeds, or with uplifted swords were leading their followers to the charge. Of course, I was surprised to find that in a real battle the officer gets in the rear of his men, as is his right and duty, that is, if his ideas of duty do not carry him so far to the rear as to make his sword useless.

The 'Rebs' forced us back by their charge, and our central lines were almost broken. The forces withdrawn from our right had taken the infantry support from our batteries, one of which, consisting of four guns, was captured. We were tired, wet, and exhausted when supports came up, and we were allowed to fall back from under the enemy's fire, but still in easy reach of the battle. I asked one of my comrades how he felt, and his reply was characteristic of the prevailing sentiment: 'I should feel like a hero if I wasn't so blank wet.' The bullets had cut queer antics among our men. A private who had a canteen of whiskey when he went into the engagement, on endeavoring to take a drink found the canteen quite empty, as a bullet had tapped it for him. Another had a part of his thumb-nail taken off. Another had a bullet pass into the toe of his boot, down between two toes, and out along the sole of his foot, without much injury. Another had a scalp wound from a bullet, which took off a strip of hair about three inches in length from the top of his head. Two of my regiment were killed outright and fourteen badly wounded, besides quite a number slightly injured. Thus I have chronicled my first day's fight, and I don't believe any of my regiment were ambitious to 'chase the enemy any farther' just at present. Refreshed with hot coffee and hard-tack, we rested from the fight, well satisfied that we had done our duty.

[...]

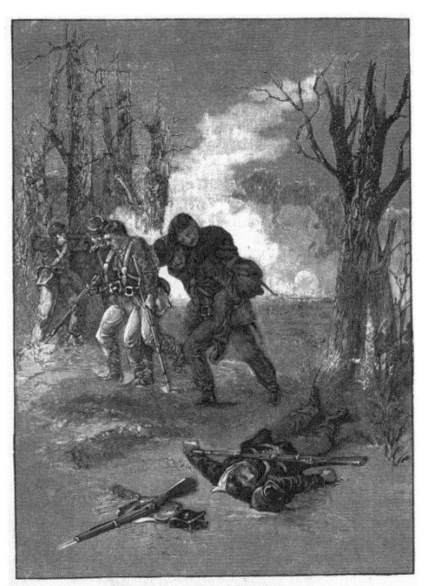

Rescuing Wounded Comrades.

Figure 18: 'Rescuing Wounded Comrades,'
from Goss, *Recollections of a Private*

Hancock's Attack [in the aftermath of the Battle of Gettysburg]

Half a dozen times the rebs stuck up something white to show that they'd got enough of fighting, and wanted to be taken in out of the wet. But others kept crowding up and taking their places as fast as we took them in. They kept the intrenchments jammed full on the other side of the logs all the time. Lively? Well, you jest bet! The rebs had to stop and throw their dead one side to get room to fight in. The logs around them were cut and slivered inter kindling-wood. Trees were cut down by bullets. The bushes and twigs were shot into flinders like broom-corn.

Our men, while sheltering their own bodies as much as possible, would reach over to shoot among the Confederates. One of my chums, with his jack-knife, enlarged a crevice in the logs so as to get a fire on them. Before he could get a chance to use it, the muzzle of a Johnnie's rifle came poking through the hole. Quick as thought, my chum, the proprietor of that port-hole, placed the muzzle of his musket against the intruding muzzle, and with a big yell fired and pushed with all his might. The suddenness of the act dislodged the reb. 'Gosh,' said my chum, grimly chuckling, 'you bet that reb was astonished!'

The spectacle was horrible in the adjacent cornfield and on the road, but in the trenches at the angle the dead men were found literally in piles. The margins of the log works were fringed with them. Thirty were counted within a distance of fifty feet.

The large number of dead on our own side who lay in this vicinity is illustrated by an incident told me by one of Wadsworth's men, belonging to the Seventy-sixth New York.

'We were moving into the fight on the morning of the 13th, when we came upon a lot of men, apparently sleeping, covered by their shelter-tents. "Why don't these men get up and go into the fight with us?" growled one of our soldiers.

'They take it mighty cool, to be sleeping under this fire!' said another, advancing towards them to make an attempt to arouse them. He kicked one with his foot, then pulled the shelter-tents from the prostrate forms, only to be appalled by the upturned, ghastly faces of dead men! 'These soldiers will never go into a fight again!' exclaimed Eggleston.

It was literally a bivouac of the dead, who had thus been hastily covered by the rough but loving hands of comrades.

The Red Badge of Courage

Stephen Crane (1871–1900) was born after the Civil War, but his most famous novel about that war was so realistic that some readers thought it was written by a veteran. *The Red Badge of Courage* was serialized in the *Philadelphia Press* in 1894 and published in book form in 1895. It was reissued in a longer version from Crane's manuscripts in 1982. Crane started the novel in 1893 after reading the 'Battles and Leaders' series in the *Century* magazine. *The Red Badge of Courage* presents an episode of the war but minimizes its historical reference. However, it has now been established that events in the novel correspond most closely with the unexpected defeat of the Union forces at the 1863 Battle of Chancellorsville in Virginia.

In Chapter 8 Henry Fleming's overwhelming impulse is to see the spectacle evoked by the sudden burst of noise from battle. When he finally does see the soldiers, the effect is grotesque from the disparate stream of images of these soldiers, an effect heightened by Crane's paragraphing. All those who pass before his wondering eyes are scarred in some way from the battle, so much so that injury has become the new norm. In contrast with the grandeur of the scenes in Fleming's imagination, there is no coherence in these sights, only a shared impulse of flight. The tattered soldier tries to engage Fleming in conversation but his innocuous enquiry about his injury reduces the youth to a panicky stammer and further flight. In a letter to John Hilliard, Crane expressed satisfaction with the reviewers' recognition of his purpose to give a 'psychological portrayal of fear.'

See also: Lee Clark Mitchell, ed., *New Essays on 'The Red Badge of Courage'* (Cambridge: Cambridge University Press, 1986); Perry Lintz, *Private Fleming at Chancellorsville: 'The Red Badge of Courage' and the Civil War* (Columbia, MO: University of Missouri Press, 2006); *Red Badge of Courage* website at http://www.redbadgeofcourage.org/; R.W. Stallman and L. Gilkes, eds, *Stephen Crane: Letters* (London: Peter Owen, 1960), p. 158.

Chapter 8

The trees began softly to sing a hymn of twilight. The sun sank until slanted bronze rays struck the forest. There was a lull in the noises of insects as if they had bowed their beaks and were making a devotional pause. There was silence save for the chanted chorus of the trees.

Then, upon this stillness, there suddenly broke a tremendous clangor of sounds. A crimson roar came from the distance.

The youth stopped. He was transfixed by this terrific medley of all noises. It was as if worlds were being rended. There was the ripping sound of musketry and the breaking crash of the artillery.

His mind flew in all directions. He conceived the two armies to be at each other panther fashion. He listened for a time. Then he began to run in the direction of the battle. He saw that it was an ironical thing for him to be running thus toward that which he had been at such pains to avoid. But he said, in substance, to himself that if the earth and the moon were about to clash, many persons would doubtless plan to get upon the roofs to witness the collision.

As he ran, he became aware that the forest had stopped its music, as if at last becoming capable of hearing the foreign sounds. The trees hushed and stood motionless. Everything seemed to be listening to the crackle and clatter and earthshaking thunder. The chorus peaked over the still earth.

It suddenly occurred to the youth that the fight in which he had been was, after all, but perfunctory popping. In the hearing of this present din he was doubtful if he had seen real battle scenes. This uproar explained a celestial battle; it was tumbling hordes a-struggle in the air.

Reflecting, he saw a sort of a humor in the point of view of himself and his fellows during the late encounter. They had taken themselves and the enemy very seriously and had imagined that they were deciding the war. Individuals must have supposed that they were cutting the letters of their names deep into everlasting tablets of brass, or enshrining their reputations forever in the hearts of their countrymen, while, as to fact, the affair would appear in printed reports under a meek and immaterial title. But he saw that it was good, else, he said, in battle every one would surely run save forlorn hopes and their ilk.

He went rapidly on. He wished to come to the edge of the forest that he might peer out.

As he hastened, there passed through his mind pictures of stupendous conflicts. His accumulated thought upon such subjects was used to form scenes. The noise was as the voice of an eloquent being, describing.

[...]

Presently he proceeded again on his forward way. The battle was like the grinding of an immense and terrible machine to him. Its complexities and powers, its grim processes, fascinated him. He must go close and see it produce corpses.

He came to a fence and clambered over it. On the far side, the ground was littered with clothes and guns. A newspaper, folded up, lay in the dirt. A dead soldier was stretched with his face hidden in his arm. Farther off there was a group of four or five corpses keeping mournful company. A hot sun had blazed upon this spot.

In this place the youth felt that he was an invader. This forgotten part of the battle ground was owned by the dead men, and he hurried, in the vague apprehension that one of the swollen forms would rise and tell him to begone.

He came finally to a road from which he could see in the distance dark and agitated bodies of troops, smoke-fringed. In the lane was a blood-stained crowd streaming to the rear. The wounded men were cursing, groaning, and wailing. In the air, always, was a mighty swell of sound that it seemed could sway the earth. With the courageous words of the artillery and the spiteful sentences of the musketry mingled red cheers. And from this region of noises came the steady current of the maimed.

One of the wounded men had a shoeful of blood. He hopped like a schoolboy in a game. He was laughing hysterically.

One was swearing that he had been shot in the arm through the commanding general's mismanagement of the army. One was marching with an air imitative of some sublime drum major. Upon his features was an unholy mixture of merriment and agony. As he marched he sang a bit of doggerel in a high and quavering voice:

> 'Sing a song 'a vic'try,
> A pocketful 'a bullets,
> Five an' twenty dead men
> Baked in a – pie.'

Parts of the procession limped and staggered to this tune.

Another had the gray seal of death already upon his face. His lips were curled in hard lines and his teeth were clinched. His hands were bloody from where he had pressed them upon his wound. He seemed to be awaiting the moment when he should pitch headlong. He stalked like the specter of a soldier, his eyes burning with the power of a stare into the unknown.

There were some who proceeded sullenly, full of anger at their wounds, and ready to turn upon anything as an obscure cause.

An officer was carried along by two privates. He was peevish. 'Don't joggle so, Johnson, yeh fool,' he cried. 'Think m' leg is made of iron? If yeh can't carry me decent, put me down an' let some one else do it.'

He bellowed at the tottering crowd who blocked the quick march of his bearers. 'Say, make way there, can't yeh? Make way, dickens take it all.'

They sulkily parted and went to the roadsides. As he was carried past they made pert remarks to him. When he raged in reply and threatened them, they told him to be damned.

The shoulder of one of the tramping bearers knocked heavily against the spectral soldier who was staring into the unknown.

The youth joined this crowd and marched along with it. The torn bodies expressed the awful machinery in which the men had been entangled.

Orderlies and couriers occasionally broke through the throng in the roadway, scattering wounded men right and left, galloping on followed by howls. The melancholy march was continually disturbed by the messengers, and sometimes by bustling batteries that came swinging and thumping down upon them, the officers shouting orders to clear the way.

There was a tattered man, fouled with dust, blood and powder stain from hair to shoes, who trudged quietly at the youth's side. He was listening with eagerness and much humility to the lurid descriptions of a bearded sergeant. His lean features wore an expression of awe and admiration. He was like a listener in a country store to wondrous tales told among the sugar barrels. He eyed the story-teller with unspeakable wonder. His mouth was agape in yokel fashion.

The sergeant, taking note of this, gave pause to his elaborate history while he administered a sardonic comment. 'Be keerful, honey, you 'll be a-ketchin' flies,' he said.

The tattered man shrank back abashed.

After a time he began to sidle near to the youth, and in a diffident way try to make him a friend. His voice was gentle as a girl's voice and his eyes were pleading. The youth saw with surprise that the soldier had two wounds, one in the head, bound with a blood-soaked rag, and the other in the arm, making that member dangle like a broken bough.

After they had walked together for some time the tattered man mustered sufficient courage to speak. 'Was pretty good fight, wa'n't it?' he timidly said. The youth, deep in thought, glanced up at the bloody and grim figure with its lamblike eyes. 'What?'

'Was pretty good fight, wa'n't it?'

'Yes,' said the youth shortly. He quickened his pace.

But the other hobbled industriously after him. There was an air of apology in his manner, but he evidently thought that he needed only to talk for a time, and the youth would perceive that he was a good fellow.

'Was pretty good fight, wa'n't it?' he began in a small voice, and the he achieved the fortitude to continue. 'Dern me if I ever see fellers fight so. Laws, how they did fight! I knowed th' boys 'd like it when they onct got square at it. Th' boys ain't had no fair chanct up t' now, but this time they showed what they was. I knowed it 'd turn out this way. Yeh can't lick them boys. No, sir! They 're fighters, they be.'

He breathed a deep breath of humble admiration. He had looked at the youth for encouragement several times. He received none, but gradually he seemed to get absorbed in his subject.

'I was talkin' 'cross pickets with a boy from Georgie, onct, an' that boy, he ses, "Your fellers 'll all run like hell when they onct hearn a gun," he ses. "Mebbe they will," I ses, "but I don't b'lieve none of it," I ses; "an' b'jiminey," I ses back t' 'um, "mebbe your fellers 'll all run like hell when they onct hearn a gun," I ses. He larfed. Well, they didn't run t' day, did they, hey? No, sir! They fit, an' fit, an' fit.'

His homely face was suffused with a light of love for the army which was to him all things beautiful and powerful.

After a time he turned to the youth. 'Where yeh hit, ol' boy?' he asked in a brotherly tone.

The youth felt instant panic at this question, although at first its full import was not borne in upon him.

'What?' he asked.

'Where yeh hit?' repeated the tattered man.

'Why,' began the youth, 'I – I – that is – why – I –'

He turned away suddenly and slid through the crowd. His brow was heavily flushed, and his fingers were picking nervously at one of his buttons. He bent his head and fastened his eyes studiously upon the button as if it were a little problem.

The tattered man looked after him in astonishment.

The Aftermath

Stephen C. Kenny (University of Liverpool)

The one undeniable truth of the American Civil War is its destruction: the appalling damage that it caused to humans, animals, and environments, to bodies, minds, relationships, families, communities, and cultures – a legacy of chaos and unmaking lasting for decades in the conflict's aftermath. All else is grist for endless debate and other volumes.

Military studies have discussed – and still do discuss – the Civil War in terms of campaigns, leadership, technological advancements, and tactical innovations. The invaluable *Library of Congress Civil War Desk Reference* (2002) has all of those steely facts for those who seek them, with sections devoted to 'Battles and the Battlefield,' 'The Armies,' and 'Weaponry.'[1] Social and cultural studies, by comparison, tend to emphasise the damage, turmoil, and suffering that the war's killing machines and deadly manoeuvres wrought. In *Living Hell: The Dark Side of the Civil War* (2014), for example, Michael C.C. Adams presents an antidote to 'romantic notions of dramatic exploits on the battlefield' by re-enacting eyewitness accounts of 'the vicious nature of combat, the terrible infliction of physical and mental wounds, the misery of soldiers living amid corpses, filth and flies [...] [And, importantly too] the many civilians who endured loss, deprivation, and violations.'[2]

The most recent scholarship on the medical dimensions of the war has drawn attention to the human health impact and the massive stimulus the

1   Margaret E. Wagner, Gary W. Gallagher, and Paul Finkelman, eds, *The Library of Congress Civil War Desk Reference* (New York: Simon and Schuster, 2002).
2   Michael C.C. Adams, *Living Hell: The Dark Side of the Civil War* (Baltimore: Johns Hopkins University Press, 2014).

conflict gave to professional medicine. In *Learning from Wounded: The Civil War and the Rise of American Medical Science* (2014), Shauna Devine counters the traditional view of medical practice in the conflict as being near medieval, exploring the making of scientific knowledge and drawing on institutional resources, including the US Army Medical Museum and the *Medical and Surgical History of the War of Rebellion*.[3] Devine's research finds abundant evidence of progress and modernisation in the medical response to the war's human slaughter. Before the war, for example, Northern medical schools complained of shortages in the human materials necessary to undertake anatomical education and research. Bloodbaths such as Antietam, Gettysburg, and Shiloh created a surplus of bodies in an instant. Across the various theatres of war, in response to Surgeon General William Hammond's Circular No. 2, doctors harvested the dead. Mutilated limbs and diseased organs were prepared, labelled, and shipped as specimens to Washington, DC, and were then catalogued and stored in the formation of the US Army Medical Museum's burgeoning collection of human remains. Circular No. 5, issued in the same moment, required case reports be submitted with human specimens and resulted in six mammoth volumes of the *Medical and Surgical History*. This landmark publication created unparalleled opportunities for knowledge production and the sharing and circulation of new scientific medical ideas and practices, offered a forum for building professional reputations and consensus, and provided graphic insights into the trials of sufferers.

Margaret Humphreys' magisterial *Marrow of Tragedy: The Health Crisis of the American Civil War* (2013) provides a peerless synthesis of Civil War medicine's history, putting particular emphasis on the role women played in caring for sick and wounded soldiers. The chaos and carnage of battles waged with muskets and cannons that obliterated flesh and bone, alongside outbreaks of deadly diseases that the swarming armies generated, demanded an immediate medical and urgent humanitarian response. The answer came in the form of swift and sometimes near painless removal of smashed and mangled limbs in improvised battlefield hospitals. Ambulance protocols were established to transport the wounded to safety behind the lines of fire. Essential supplies and care packages filled with food and clothing were delivered from the home front by the Sanitary Commission. Then there were the caring strangers, the volunteer nurses who tended the wounded

3   Shauna Devine, *Learning from the Wounded: The Civil War and the Rise of American Medical Science* (Chapel Hill, NC: University of North Carolina Press, 2014); Joseph K. Barnes, ed., *The Medical and Surgical History of the War of Rebellion* (Washington, DC: US Government Printing Office, 1870–88).

thousands in massive general hospitals such as Richmond's Chimborazo and Philadelphia's Satterlee.[4]

Another form of medical response and progress born of tragedy came with the companies that emerged to supply disabled veterans with artificial limbs and other prosthetic devices. Politicians either side of the Mason–Dixon line seized upon empty sleeves and trouser legs as symbols of heroism and valour, while limbless ex-soldiers sought practical means of rehabilitation and reintegration into the worlds of work and society. In *Mending Broken Soldiers* (2012), Guy R. Hasegawa examines both the Union and Confederate programs to supply injured veterans with prosthetic devices and the growing industry of providers – such as Hanger, Palmer, and Salem – that met this desperate need. Hasegawa's research features testimony from some of the grateful recipients of artificial limbs, but we still await a broader social history of disability experiences following the war.[5]

Dead and damaged bodies had profound consequences for American society both during the war and for the years that followed. The war was an absolute disaster for humanity, slaying more than a million Americans in battle, or by disease, with many thousands more suffering devastating injuries and painful losses. Historian and Harvard president Drew Gilpin Faust's bestselling *This Republic of Suffering: Death and the American Civil War* (2008) examined how the colossal carnage of the Civil War utterly transformed the American culture of death.[6] The new methods of killing, executed in battles fought far from home, near obliterated the antebellum era's cherished ideal of a 'Good Death' among friends and family. Soldiers' bodies could be shredded and utterly anonymised by new and deadly weapons, or stripped of identity by battlefield scavengers, left abandoned and tragically Unknown, with hundreds of thousands of men on both sides dying without hope of recognition. Faust highlights the various responses to the growing problem of war death, seen, for example, in the establishment of national military cemeteries, such as Gettysburg, the rise of the funeral industry, the commodification of death, and in new cultures of mourning – the most elaborate of which became the post-bellum South's cult of the Confederacy's Lost Cause.

4   Margaret Humphreys, *Marrow of Tragedy: The Health Crisis of the American Civil War* (Baltimore: The Johns Hopkins University Press, 2013).
5   Guy R. Hasegawa, *Mending Broken Soldiers: The Union and Confederate Program to Supply Artificial Limbs* (Carbondale, IL: Southern Illinois University Press, 2012).
6   Drew Gilpin Faust, *This Republic of Suffering: Death and the American Civil War* (New York: Vintage Books, 2008).

Stephen Berry's inspirational collection *Weirding the War: Stories from the Civil War's Ragged Edges* (2011) thoroughly reconsiders the war's traumatic impacts using a number of innovative new approaches and uncommon sources, including coroners' reports, material culture, the ruined landscape, a focus on Southern female responses to amputated soldiers, and wartime hunger. Building on Eric T. Dean, Jr.'s pioneering work *Shook Over Hell: Post-Traumatic Stress, Vietnam, and the Civil War* (1997), Diane Miller Sommerville's essay in Berry's volume blends medical records, memoirs, and newspaper reports to explore the dual burden of psychological damage suffered by Confederate veterans – war trauma and then return to a defeated 'nation' – reflecting on how this damage shaped the post-war South. Sommerville and others in Berry's excellent edited volume make the important point that the war's traumatic impact needs to be extended to include the partners and families of soldier survivors, as well as the communities that often struggled to realize their reintegration.[7]

There were over 200,000 African Americans in the Union forces – 10,000 of those were sailors, but the majority were soldiers. Yet images that captured the labour of burial parties deployed in the wake of battles reveal that white assumptions of black inferiority consigned many African American volunteers to the most dismal and onerous forms of labour. In a valuable digression from her magnum opus on the war's medical dimensions, Margaret Humphreys produced *Intensely Human: The Health of the Black Soldier in the American Civil War* (2008), and uncovered the broader story of how white racism shaped the soldiering, health, and medical experiences of African Americans troops in the Union Army. While professional medicine was most fully racialized in the South under slavery, in the North white physicians used the recruitment process to test racial theories and as an opportunity to dissect bodies in pursuit of what they saw as the mystery of black distinctiveness.[8] Jim Downs' innovative work, *Sick from Freedom: African-American Illness and Suffering during the Civil War and Reconstruction* (2012), tells another new story about medical racism, using records from the Medical Division of the Freedmen's Bureau to highlight the continuing struggle for health faced by newly freed

---

7   Stephen Berry, ed., *Weirding the War: Stories from the Civil War's Ragged Edges* (Athens, GA: University of Georgia Press, 2011); Eric T. Dean, Jr., *Shook Over Hell: Post-Traumatic Stress, Vietnam, and the Civil War* (Cambridge, MA: Harvard University Press, 1997).

8   Margaret Humphreys, *Intensely Human: The Health of the Black Soldier in the American Civil War* (Baltimore: Johns Hopkins University Press, 2008).

slaves caught up in the epidemiological disaster produced by the Civil War and Reconstruction.[9]

As distant witnesses to the war and its victims, readers have to work hard not to wallow in the appalling details of its dark archive and see some way forward. Once viewed, remembered, and consumed – then what? This companion volume offers a raw record of bones and corpses strewn across scarred battlefields. Uncanny clinical images of the severely wounded before and after treatment and prosthetic devices rework our understanding of the body, and the heightened language of memoirs and fictions strain to recall a kaleidoscope of emotions in the midst of war's crimson mayhem. This is still the war's aftermath and we are still trying to make sense of it.

9   Jim Downs, *Sick from Freedom: African-American Illness and Suffering during the Civil War and Reconstruction* (Oxford and New York: Oxford University Press, 2012).

Contributors

Dillon Carroll is a PhD candidate at the University of Georgia. He is finishing a dissertation that explores mental illness among veterans of the American Civil War, and how families and society absorbed and compensated for that damage. He currently lives and works in New York City.

Robert Leigh Davis is a Professor in the Department of English at Wittenberg University, in Springfield, Ohio. His publications include *Whitman and the Romance of Medicine*.

Mick Gidley is an Emeritus Professor of American Literature and Culture in the School of English at the University of Leeds. He is writing a cultural history of the photography of E.O. Hoppe. His recent books include *Photography and the USA*, *Edward S. Curtis and the North American Indian Project in the Field*, and (as editor) *Writing with Light: Words and Photographs in American Texts*.

Susan-Mary Grant is a Professor of American History and Deputy Head in the School of History, Classics and Archaeology at Newcastle University. Her publications include *The War for a Nation: The American Civil War*.

Stephen C. Kenny is a Lecturer in Nineteenth- and Twentieth-Century North American History in the Department of History at the University of Liverpool. He has published essays exploring human experiments under American slavery in *Endeavour*, *Social History of Medicine*, the *Journal of the History of Medicine and Allied Sciences*, and the *Bulletin of the History of Medicine*. He is currently completing a monograph titled *Dark Medicine: Racism, Power and the Culture of American Slavery*.

Shaun Lowndes is an illustrator based in Manchester, England. He has been producing artwork for the past 30 years exploring themes of masculinity. His recent collection of images – including 'The Homecoming' – examines the lives and losses of the men, women, and children of the American Civil War.

Angel Martin is a digital cyberpunk artist. Angel's work looks at historical events with a pan-dimensional twist. If you think of a photograph as a moment frozen in time, Angel's work questions the idea of time as linear, twisting perceptions by moving technology out of sequence creating alternative realities. You can see more of Angel's work at http://badangel.artweb.com.

David Seed is Emeritus Professor of American Literature in the English Department at the University of Liverpool. His publications include *American Travelers in Liverpool* and (as editor with Susan Castillo) *American Travel and Empire*. He is currently working on a project about nuclear terrorism in the wake of 9/11.

Chris Williams is the Research and Knowledge Exchange Impact Officer in the Faculty of Humanities and Social Sciences at the University of Liverpool. He is currently researching a history of Abercromby Square in Liverpool.

Select Bibliography

Adams, George Worthington, *Doctors in Blue: The Medical History of the Union Army in the Civil War*, 2nd edn (Baton Rouge, LA: Louisiana State University Press, 1996).

Adams, Michael C.C., *Living Hell: The Dark Side of the Civil War* (Baltimore: Johns Hopkins University Press, 2014).

Barton, Michael, and Larry M. Logue, eds, *The Civil War Soldier: A Historical Reader* (New York: New York University Press, 2002).

Berry, Stephen, ed., *Weirding the War: Stories from the Civil War's Ragged Edges* (Athens, GA: University of Georgia Press, 2011).

Blight, David W., *Race and Reunion: The Civil War in American Memory* (Cambridge, MA: Belknap Press, 2003).

Bollet, Alfred Jay, *Civil War Medicine: Challenges and Triumphs* (Tucson, AZ: Galen Press, 2002).

Burns, Stanley B., *Shooting Soldiers: Civil War Medical Photography by R.B. Bontecou* (New York: Burns Archive Press, 2011).

Clarke, Frances M., *War Stories: Suffering and Sacrifice in the Civil War North* (Chicago: University of Chicago Press, 2011).

Clinton, Caroline, ed., *Battle Scars: Gender and Sexuality in the American Civil War* (New York: Oxford University Press, 2006).

Clinton, Caroline, ed., *Divided Houses: Gender and the Civil War* (New York: Oxford University Press, 1992).

Cullen, Jim, *The Civil War in Popular Culture: A Reusable Past* (Washington, DC: The Smithsonian Institution, 1995).

Cullen-Sizer, Lyde, and Jim Cullen, eds, *The Civil War Era: An Anthology of Sources* (Oxford: Wiley-Blackwell, 2005).

Cunningham, H.H., *Doctors in Gray: The Confederate Medical Service* (Baton Rouge, LA: Louisiana State University Press, 1993).

Damman, Gordon, and Alfred Jay Bollet, *Images of Civil War Medicine: A Photographic History* (New York: Demos Health Publishing, 2007).

Davis, Keith F. "'A Terrible Distinctness': Photography of the Civil War Era", in Martha A. Sandweiss, ed., *Photography in Nineteenth-Century America*. New York: Harry N. Abrams for Amon Carter Museum, 1991), pp. 128–79.

Denney, Robert E., *Civil War Medicine: Care and Comfort of the Wounded* (New York: Sterling Publishing, 1994).

Devine, Shauna, *Learn from the Wounded: The Civil War and the Rise of American Medical Science* (Chapel Hill, NC: University of North Carolina Press, 2014).

Fahs, Alice, *The Imagined Civil War: Popular Literature of the North and South, 1861–1865* (Chapel Hill, NC: University of North Carolina Press, 2001).

Fahs, Alice, and Joan Waugh, eds, *The Memory of the Civil War in American Culture* (Chapel Hill, NC: University of North Carolina Press, 2004).

Faust, Drew Gilpin, *This Republic of Suffering: Death and the American Civil War* (New York: Alfred A. Knopf, 2008).

Flannery, Michael, *Civil War Pharmacy: A History of Drugs, Drug Supply and Provision, and Therapeutics for the Union and Confederacy* (Boca Raton, FL: CRC Press, 2004).

Foreman, Amanda, *A World on Fire: Britain's Crucial Role in the American Civil War* (New York: Random House, 2012).

Frassanito, William A. *Antietam: The Photographic Legacy of America's Bloodiest Day*. New York: Charles Scribner's Sons, 1978.

Frassanito, William A. *Gettysburg: A Journey in Time*. New York: Scribner's Sons, 1975.

Freemon, Frank R., *Gangrene and Glory: Medical Care during the American Civil War* (Urbana, IL: University of Illinois Press, 2001).

Grant, Susan-Mary, *The War for a Nation: The American Civil War* (London and New York: Routledge, 2006).

Grant, Susan-Mary, and Peter J. Parish, eds, *Legacy of Disunion: The Enduring Significance of the American Civil War* (Baton Rouge, LA: Louisiana State University Press, 2003).

Humphreys, Margaret, *Marrow of Tragedy: The Health Crisis of the American Civil War* (Baltimore: Johns Hopkins University Press, 2013).

Kreiser, Lawtence A., Jr., and Randal Allred, eds, *The Civil War in Popular Culture: Memory and Meaning* (Lexington, KY: University Press of Kentucky, 2014).

Lande, R. Gregory, *Madness, Malingering and Malfeasance: The Transformation of Psychiatry and the Law in the Civil War Era* (Washington, DC: Brassey's US, 2005).

Logue, Larry M., and Michael Barton, eds, *The Civil War Veteran: A Historical Reader* (New York: New York University Press, 2007).

Masur, Louis P., ed., *The Real War Will Never Get in the Books: Selections from Writers during the Civil War* (New York: Oxford University Press, 1993).

McPherson, James M., and Steven E. Woodworth, eds, *The American Civil War: A Handbook of Literature and Research* (Westport, CT: Greenwood Publishing, 1996).

Miller, Brian Craig, *Empty Sleeves: Amputation in the Civil War South* (Athens, GA: University of Georgia Press, 2015).

Miller, Francis Trevelyan, *The Photographic History of the Civil War*, 10 vols (New York: Review of Reviews, 1911–12).

Nelson, Megan Kate, *Ruin Nation: Destruction and the American Civil War* (Athens, GA: University of Georgia Press, 2012).

Rosenheim, Jeff L., *Photography and the American Civil War* (New York: Metropolitan Museum of Art, 2013).

Rutkow, Ira, *Bleeding Blue and Gray: Civil War Surgery and the Evolution of American Medicine* (New York: Random House, 2005).

Samuels, Shirley, *Facing America: Iconography and the Civil War* (New York: Oxford University Press, 2004).

Savage, Douglas J., *Civil War Medicine* (New York: Chelsea House, 2000).

Schmidt, James M., and Guy R. Hasegawa, eds, *Years of Change and Suffering: Modern Perspectives on Civil War Medicine* (Roseville, MN: Edinborough Press, 2010).

Schroeder-Lein, Glenna R., *The Encyclopedia of Civil War Medicine* (London and New York: Routledge, 2008).

Schulz, Jane E., *Women at the Front: Hospital Workers in Civil War America* (Chapel Hill, NC: University of North Carolina Press, 1997).

Sheehan, Tanya, *Doctored: The Medicine of Photography in Nineteenth-century America* (University Park, PA: Pennsylvania University Press, 2011).

Smith, Mark M., *The Smell of Battle, the Taste of Siege: A Sensory History of the Civil War* (New York: Oxford University, 2014).

Straubing, Harold Elk, *In Hospital and Camp: The Civil War through the Eyes of its Doctors and Nurses* (Mechanicsburg, PA: Stackpole Books, 1993).

Thompson, Meg, *The Aftermath of Battle: The Burial of the Civil War Dead* (El Dorado Hills, CA: Savas Beatie, 2015).

Wilbur, C. Keith, *Civil War Medicine* (Guilford, CT: Globe Pequot Press, 1998).

Journals, etc.

'Civil War Diaries and Letters,' *DIY History*, University of Iowa Libraries, at http://diyhistory.lib.uiowa.edu/collections/show/8.

Civil War History, Kent State University Press.

Civil War Journal, A&E television documentary series, 1993–98.

Civil War Primary Documents, Personal Diaries, Journals, Letters, Cartoons, Art, Images, Poetry, Literature & Music, at http://www.teacheroz.com/Civil_War_Documents.htm.

Civil War Regiments: A Journal of the American Civil War (1991–2001).

Civil War Times, Welder Historical Group.

Journal of Civil War Medicine, Society of Civil War Surgeons.

Journal of the Civil War Era, University of North Carolina Press.

Life and Limb: The Toll of the American Civil War, US National Library of Medicine, at http://www.nlm.nih.gov/exhibition/lifeandlimb/index.html. The library also has an extensive digital archive.

Index